CAN I SPEAK TO THE HORMONE LADY?

Managing Menopause and Hormone Imbalances

Jeannie Collins Beaudin

Can I Speak to the Hormone Lady?

While every precaution has been taken in the preparation of this book, the publisher and author assume no responsibility for errors or omissions, or for damages resulting from the use of the information contained herein. All treatment decisions should be carefully discussed with your personal physician.

Jeannie Collins Beaudin
Visit my website at www.jeanniebeaudin.wixsite.com/author

First Edition: February 2019
Collins Pharmacy Ltd.

ISBN-978-1-79-769135-0

CONTENTS

INTRODUCTION

WHAT'S THIS BOOK ABOUT?

I wrote this book to educate women about the many choices available for treatment of menopausal symptoms, and which ones have lower side effects and risk. And I wrote it to help women learn the signs and symptoms that tell them what hormones are missing or out of balance. My ultimate goal is to enable women to better understand their bodies, what has gone wrong, their options for treatment, and how to clearly communicate what they need to their health care providers.

There are many general books on menopause. This book is for the woman who wants to know more than the basics. I spent many years searching for information in published texts, at international conferences, and in scientific studies. And I learned an immense amount from and for the hundreds of women I counseled in my pharmacy practice to help them find relief from their hormone-related symptoms. When I retired from active pharmacy practice, I wanted to continue to help women have an easier passage through menopause and other times of hormone imbalance. I decided to capture all I'd learned in a form that could be used by women and the health professionals who help them make treatment decisions. I wrote this book about hormones, menopause, and how to diagnose and fix problems that occur when hormones are not in the correct balance.

In Can I Speak to the Hormone Lady, I explain various treatments, from natural products to prescription hormones, and how these fit together. Because natural (or "bioidentical") hormones were a specialty for my compounding pharmacy practice that I studied for over 10 years, I also include detailed information about how these are different from standard hormones and how they are prescribed. I describe how a woman's body responds to changing levels of hormones, and the signs that tell us what hormones are missing. And I explain why I am convinced that the best approach to treating menopause symptoms, if hormones are needed, is to replace only missing hormones, use the same hormones as those our bodies make, use lowest effective dose and avoid administering them through the digestive system.

As a pharmacist, I used my knowledge of hormone actions and available treatments to create individualized treatments for women who were not receiving adequate relief through other health care channels. Most of the women I counseled had very challenging symptoms. But I found that taking time for a detailed discussion and truly focusing on her individual problems, needs and preferences was the best way to create an ideal treatment program for her.

Since doctors are trained to look for scientific evidence, but often are not familiar with studies that have been done with alternative treatments, I have added references in this book to studies that support some of the lesser-known treatments, just as I did in reports I sent to doctors on my clients' behalf.

I believe that an ideal menopause treatment should consider all of a woman's complaints plus her preferences for addressing them. It should create a customized plan to improve her life. Unfortunately, with the health system we have, many doctors cannot take the time they need to review all of a woman's hormone related symptoms.

However, you can learn to analyze your symptoms yourself and be prepared to concisely explain to your doctor what problems you are experiencing and the impact they are having in your life, as well as the treatment you are interested in trying.

No one knows your body, your preferences and your needs better than yourself. I believe that any therapy should be an informed collaboration between you and the health care professionals that you trust. Informed collaboration means that you receive adequate information to understand what is happening in your body, you are told what treatment options are available to you and the pros and cons of each, and you have a say in what treatment you receive.

And, included in the information that you are given, should be sources that inform you of what you can do yourself to take charge of the problem you are trying to correct. Having a sense of control of treatment choice is considered a positive factor in improving your health and is more likely to result in a treatment that you will want to use.

Non-drug therapy ideas that will help you live a healthier lifestyle abound on the internet, and you may have read some of these sources. But keep in mind, although there is almost too much information on the Internet to digest, there is plenty of misinformation as well. One good rule of thumb I have learned is to be skeptical when a site is giving you information and also trying to sell you something. Bias is a critical factor that we all need to be aware of, even in scientific research, where the information can be explained in a way favorable to the sponsor of the study or a product they are trying to sell. This problem is even more significant on the Internet where information is much less regulated. Ideal sites to look for are those sponsored by an educational institution, government or large health institution.

I have made a conscious effort in the writing of this book, to present a completely unbiased discussion of treatments that are available. My experiences, as a pharmacist who has studied standard medicines, alternatives and natural remedies, combined with the experience gained by helping many women to improve their lives, has given me a different point of view than most health professionals. Being completely retired now, I have no potential to gain from "selling" this information other than the sale of the book itself and the joy of having shared what I have learned with a broader audience. I hope that many women will benefit from the information I have presented here.

In addition to information on menopause and its treatment, I also include the system I used to analyze hormone levels and imbalances using symptoms and changes over time. You will find the worksheet I used with hundreds of women, along with a detailed explanation of how to interpret the results. I also walk you through how to discuss your analysis and preferences with your doctor. The focus of this book is to educate and empower women like you to become involved in their choice of menopause treatment.

I would also like you to realize that, if you don't feel comfortable doing this yourself, you can ask a specialty pharmacist or naturopathic doctor to help you assess your individual needs and preferences. These health professionals can more easily schedule the time needed to thoroughly assess all of your symptoms. They can also communicate these to your physician on your behalf.

But I firmly believe that any woman can understand how her body functions and the signs and symptoms that tell her what is happening within. You simply need to learn and observe the monthly hormone-related patterns in your body, watching for subtle (or not so subtle!) changes, and understand what these changes are telling you.

CHAPTER ONE

HOW CAN I REDUCE MENOPAUSE SYMPTOMS?

I like to think of menopause treatment as a series of "levels". You should always consider the lowest level treatment first and only advance to the next step if it is necessary for control of symptoms. With medications, "less is more"... a person is always better off taking the lowest level and lowest dose of treatment that will work for them. Especially with hormones, you should always take the lowest amount that will provide the relief you need.

The stepwise levels of treatment I consider when helping a woman to control symptoms related to the menopausal change include:

1. Exercise, diet, lifestyle changes,
2. Herbal medications, nutritional supplements,
3. Low dose hormones the same as the body produces, and
4. Pharmaceutical hormones, that are chemically different and generally stronger than our natural hormones.

Level 1: Exercise, Diet, Lifestyle Changes

The first level of treatment includes exercise, improving diet, and making healthy changes in your lifestyle. These are changes all women should make to feel more comfortable and improve their health in the future.

Exercise can help to even hormone production and, since it also helps to reduce circulating stress hormones, can be useful in women who notice their symptoms are worse during and after stressful situations.

Stress hormones, which produce your "fight or flight" reaction, set you up for exercise - speeding your heart rate, increasing your blood pressure and blood sugar, and more - and exercise works to reverse these effects. Exercise improves health in many other ways too. As little as 30 minutes of moderate exercise 3 times a week can improve your health. Building exercise into your daily routine works too - it doesn't need to be a session at the gym. Take the stairs, park in the far corner unless it's pouring rain... look for ways to add more movement to your day, wherever possible. Ten minutes 3 times a day is considered equal to a 30-minute session.

Eating more vegetables can help to even out your own hormone levels to a certain extent as well. This is because many vegetables contain plant-based hormones, also called "phytohormones". When hormone levels are very low, these weak phytohormones can exert a small hormone-like effect. When natural hormone levels surge, phytohormones can have a dulling effect, reducing natural hormone action by competing with your own stronger hormones.

Here is a simple piece of diet advice I stumbled across: serve your plate with ¾ vegetables and ¼ meat and have 5 different colors of food in each meal. Different colors of food tend to contain different nutrients, so a variety of colors on your plate will help make sure you are getting what you need to stay healthy. I often like to quote author, Michael Pollan's, Food Rules:

- Eat food (real food, not processed)
- Mostly plants and
- Not too much

Dress in layers that are easy to remove and install a ceiling fan over your bed to improve your comfort and your sleep if you are suffering from hot flashes. The faster you can cool yourself when your brain's temperature regulation setting drops, the less time the hot flash tends to last and the less discomfort you will experience.

These general "level 1" improvements and others along these lines are good for any woman experiencing a hormone change to consider. Small changes can add together to make a significant improvement and can add to any higher level therapy you may need to consider. As well, these are all healthy changes. Your reproductive years are becoming part of your past and you want to look forward to a healthy and happy retirement doing things you've always wanted to do. It's a goodtime to consider what you can do to stay healthy and active as you age gracefully. The effort to make these changes is an excellent investment in your future lifestyle.

Level 2: Herbal Medicines and Nutritional Supplements

The second level of menopause treatments includes herbal medications and nutritional supplements. I'm not a fan of taking a lot of supplements, but you might benefit from targeted ones. The two herbal medicines I have found most useful with my clients are black cohosh and vitex (also called chaste berry). Some women find good relief from hot flashes with black cohosh alone, but others respond better to a combination product that contains both ingredients (usually with others added). Herbal combinations are available from several reputable companies and are much simpler and less expensive to take than buying each ingredient separately.

Black cohosh is rich in phytohormones, so helps to regulate swings in estrogen levels in the same manner as plant foods, but with more noticeable results. Vitex helps to increase the effect of a second major hormone, progesterone, creating improved hormone balance. I suspect that the women who benefited more from the combination products needed a progesterone boost as well as the black cohosh phytoestrogen effect. I have also had perimenopausal clients with heavy menstrual flow (a sign of low progesterone in relation to the amount of estrogen being produced) report normalizing of their periods after starting vitex.

Nutritional supplements can also be helpful for menopause symptoms. Magnesium is one I have often recommended to improve sleep when taken at bedtime. Magnesium tends to relax muscles and cause drowsiness, especially if it is lacking in the diet. One study I read suggested that as many as 30% of diets in North America are lacking in magnesium, as this mineral is often removed during food processing. A supplement taken at bedtime will sometimes help improve sleep and, since you also need magnesium for healthy bones, you might benefit from this supplement in more than one way! Also, magnesium is absorbed better if taken away from meals so taking it at bedtime makes sense regardless of the reason you are taking it. Note that it can cause diarrhea if too high a dose is taken. If you notice a trend toward loose stools, reduce the dose or stop taking it completely. As magnesium is cleared by the kidney, those with chronic kidney disease tend to be less tolerant of magnesium supplements.

Another supplement I have found useful for addressing sleep problems associated with stress is pantothenic acid or vitamin B5. Waking in the middle of the night with your mind racing and unable to return to sleep in spite of being exhausted, suggests a nighttime spike in production of stress hormones - hormones that should remain low during the night. Pantothenic acid can help prevent these inappropriate spikes in production, improving your sleep. I usually suggest taking 100mg at bedtime if waking occurs in the middle of the night, or at supper time for stressed people who have trouble falling asleep. Combination B-Complex vitamins all contain some vitamin B5. You will note that some vitamin B combinations are labeled as "stress formulas" and these are safe and well worth trying for minor anxiety symptoms or difficulty sleeping.

Of course, there are many herbal and nutritional supplements that can be helpful, and you may want to consult with a naturopath or knowledgeable pharmacist for expert one-on-one advice. However, avoid getting caught up in taking a lot of different supplements and herbal medicines. As with prescription medicines, the more you take, the greater the chance of interactions and side effects. I generally suggest a trial of one month with a supplement and, if you don't notice an improvement, don't continue taking it.

Level 3: Low Dose Hormones

If you have severe symptoms of hormone imbalance, or herbal medications haven't helped, there's a good chance you would benefit from directly supplementing the missing hormone(s).

Bioidentical hormones (or hormones that are "biologically identical" to those produced by your body) are available in different forms and strengths. They can be taken by mouth, suppository, through the skin or under the tongue. Some forms are available commercially, and some need to be compounded or "made from scratch" by a pharmacist.

The goals of bioidentical hormone replacement therapy (BHRT) are to:

- Correct problematic imbalances using hormones identical to those we produce,
- Replace only the missing hormones,
- Time administration to mimic normal hormone secretion and
- Use a dose that will provide a normal blood level for the current stage of life.

Of course, the ultimate goal is to help women feel better without side effects or increased risk of disease.

We are always adding to a woman's own production, so the amount needed will vary from person to person; as well, the amount that is "normal" can vary from woman to woman. Great emphasis is placed on balancing progesterone and estrogen, and on looking at the entire hormone picture. By analyzing a wide range of symptoms, we screen for all of the main reproductive hormones: the estrogens, progesterone and testosterone. Ideally thyroid and adrenal hormones should also be considered as they can influence the reproductive hormones as well as have a negative impact on how a woman feels if not being produced in the normal amounts and timing. We also strive to use the lowest dose of hormones that will improve symptoms satisfactorily.

Availability

Many forms of bioidentical hormones are compounded to customize the content, dose or dosage form. Note that pharmaceutical compounding means preparation of a personalized medicine from individual ingredients by a pharmacist, according to a doctor's prescription. Although simply mixing any two substances together is considered compounding, it can also involve making a medicinal product completely from basic ingredients, offering complete control of the content and form. Because of the similarity to baking, we sometimes simply refer to compounding as "making a product from scratch", borrowing the term often used in the kitchen.

But commercial BHRT is available also. The bioidentical estrogen, estradiol, is available in tablets, patches, vaginal rings and vaginal suppositories. The bioidentical progestogen, progesterone, is manufactured in capsules and vaginal gel. It is also available commercially as a cream in some countries. Most commercial testosterone products are manufactured for men and are ten to fifty times stronger than a normal dose a woman would use.

It is important to use an identical human hormone because any change in the molecule can alter one or more of its actions, as I will explain in more detail later. Hormones act at many different sites in the body and, while researchers may observe the desired action in the tissue being examined, a non-identical hormone may have an effect different from the human hormone elsewhere, creating a side effect or negative consequence that may not be detected for years.

Bioidentical hormone replacement therapy, or BHRT, and its advantages will be discussed more throughout this book.

Level 4: Pharmaceutical Hormones

I refer to hormones that are not the same as your body makes as "pharmaceutical hormones".

If you are considering pharmaceutical hormones or birth control pills for treatment of menopause symptoms, level 4 of my treatment choices, you need to carefully weigh the pros and cons... These hormones, that are different from those produced by our bodies, are the strongest therapy option and one I rarely recommend for menopause symptoms, as bioidentical hormones are a better choice, in my opinion, and work well to relieve symptoms. At one time experts seemed to believe that if hormones "kept you young" then the more, the better! However, now we know that too much hormone activity can be as problematic as too little, and recommended dosages have steadily decreased over the years.

Original doses of an early hormone therapy, Premarin (conjugated equine estrogen or CEE), were as high as 2.5mg daily and it was taken alone. With use, it was noted that the endometrial lining of the uterus became thickened, and risk of cancer in this area was increased. Doses were reduced to 0.625mg and a second hormone, medroxyprogesterone, was added to prevent endometrial growth. This regimen worked very well to reverse the endometrial cancer risk. Several studies were done with the 0.625mg tablets that suggested it lowered risk factors for other diseases of aging so, although a lower 0.3mg tablet became available, it was not often prescribed as the effects of that strength weren't well enough "proven". However, I suspect that the 0.3mg dosage would have been enough for many women and negative effects may have been reduced.

While researching another issue years ago, I stumbled across studies on medroxyprogesterone dating back to the early 1990s suggesting it might increase risk of breast cancer. However, about the same time, another study by the World Health Organization failed to identify an increased risk of this cancer. So, its use continued until the landmark Women's Health Initiative (WHI) study found clear evidence of more overall risk than benefit from the combination therapy of CEE and medroxyprogesterone, including an increased risk of breast cancer. These results caused the study to be stopped in 2002, earlier than scheduled. Stopping a study early gets the attention of the science community and the media, and most doctors stopped prescribing both hormone preparations right away.

Newer research and reanalysis of the data from the Women's Health Initiative Study suggest that hormone risks were not as severe as stated in 2002, especially in women within 10 years of menopause. There has been a gradual return to using hormones particularly in women who have not found relief with other therapies. However, all sources recommend using hormones only for treating menopause symptoms (not for prevention of chronic diseases), using the lowest effective dose for the shortest time needed, and generally not taking them for more than 5 to 7 years. Some sources suggest as little as 2 years.

When it comes to pharmaceutical hormones there are many different varieties, a number of which are used for birth control. With all these different "cousins" of our own hormones, there are subtle differences in their actions and side effects because of the differences in their structure. There has also been a gradual reduction in the strength of birth control pills being introduced over the years. These factors have made it difficult to analyze the effects of long-term hormone use in women, especially with most birth control pills and menopausal hormone replacement regimens being combinations and a variety of different hormones.

In general, however, birth control pills have been found to be associated with reduced risk of endometrial and ovarian cancers, and with increased risk of breast, cervical and liver cancers. They are generally not recommended in women over 35 who smoke or who have heart disease, high blood pressure, diabetes or blood clots, due to added risk from the hormones in these pills.

In spite of this, doctors will sometimes prescribe low dose birth control pills to women in perimenopause (the years before periods stop when women are experiencing various hormone changes and symptoms) to control menopause symptoms as well as to prevent pregnancy. This may be a good option if you need birth control and don't have any of the cautions listed above, but it's a "one size fits all" approach that, in my experience, only addresses some symptoms a woman may be experiencing.

For a significant number of women, perimenopause is characterized by lowered production of progesterone and normal or increased production of estrogen, with classic symptoms of heavier menstrual flow and skipped periods. While the synthetic progestin in the birth control pill generally will control the heavy periods, the extra estrogen is certainly not needed at a time when natural estrogen production is often higher than normal, creating a different set of excess estrogen effects for these women that can include weight gain and fluid retention.

In contrast, the approach I used (and that of other pharmacists and naturopaths who do similar hormone analysis) offers assessment of symptoms to determine which hormones are missing and makes an effort to replace only those hormones.

Some practitioners use saliva or blood hormone tests to assess or confirm what hormones are being over or under produced, and choose a therapy based on this information.

CHAPTER TWO

A SHORT HISTORY OF HORMONE THERAPY...

Hormone therapy isn't new. In my reading, I learned that, in ancient times, the hormone-rich urine of teenagers was collected, dried and used on the skin as a hormone supplement. Using urine for its hormone content is not the most appetizing thought, but this is essentially how the hormone supplement, Premarin, is made. Urine from pregnant horses, rich in estrogens, is collected and the hormones it contains are processed into pills.

Problems with estrogen-only therapy

Initially, estrogen was the only hormone researchers believed women needed to address as they went through menopause. Estrogen would keep women young, vibrant and sexy. It would stop hot flashes and keep women healthier as they aged. As mentioned earlier, after several years, it was observed that women taking estrogen alone were at higher risk of developing uterine cancer. I'll explain what happened, and how it affected treatment for menopause symptoms.

In a normal cycle, our own hormone, progesterone, balances the effect of estrogen on the uterus and prevents an increased cancer risk. Researchers had developed a process to make progesterone inexpensively in a lab in 1935, but this process was never patented. Anyone could copy the process and create their own progesterone product.

Another factor was the fact that progesterone, when taken by mouth, was immediately broken down by the liver. Pills were believed to be preferred by most women, so this was another reason to create an alternative for progesterone - one that would be absorbed more easily when taken by mouth.

So, researchers added a "medroxy" group onto the progesterone molecule, creating medroxyprogesterone. This made the hormone less recognizable to body systems, so it was not broken down as soon as it was absorbed from the stomach. It was active when taken as a pill, and it worked as well as progesterone to protect the uterus from extra estrogen women were taking for their menopause symptoms.

Product patents may have had an influence

Of course, being an entirely new molecule, the newly invented medroxyprogesterone was patentable. Having a patent for medroxyprogesterone made it more profitable for the manufacturer, because patent laws protected them from competition... an additional reason to promote the use of a synthetic alternative to progesterone.

As a result, Medroxyprogesterone became part of the standard Premarin hormone replacement therapy instead of progesterone.

I want to note that a progesterone capsule has since been developed that allows about 10% of the hormone in it to bypass breakdown by the liver and reach the circulation. Progesterone is mixed with peanut oil that binds tightly to it, protecting about 10% from being changed into breakdown products as soon as it is absorbed. However, the other 90% that is changed causes side effects of drowsiness and dizziness that many women find objectionable. And, of course, anyone with a peanut allergy would need to avoid this product.

Changes can cause side effects

One side effect of medroxyprogesterone, however, is breast soreness, whereas natural progesterone acts to prevent breast soreness caused by excess estrogen. This suggests the addition of the "medroxy" group changed the part of the progesterone molecule that acts in the breast. It is now known that medroxyprogesterone's stimulation of breast cells not only results in breast soreness, but it can increase the risk of breast cancer. Studies dating back as far as 1989 have suggested this increase in risk.1 2 Natural progesterone, on the other hand, is believed by many clinicians to have a protective effect on the breast,3 although more study should be done to prove this. A study by K Chang and

---

[1] . Depot medroxyprogesterone (Depo-Provera) and risk of breast cancer.BMJ 1989;299:759. http://dx.doi.org/10.1136/bmj.299.6702.759

[2] . Li Cl,Beaber EF, et al, Cancer Res. 2012 Apr 15'72(8):2028-35, Effect of depo-medroxyprogesterone acetate on breast cancer risk among women 20 to 44 years of age.

[3] . Pike MC et al, Epidemiologic Reviews. 1993;15(1).17-35.

his colleagues in 1995 showed that adding progesterone to an estrogen cream applied to the breast resulted in a reduced rate of cell division, as compared to an increased rate of cell division when an estrogen-only cream was applied.[4] Like endometrial cells, an increased rate of cell division in breast cells is understood to create an increased chance of error in cell division, and more errors increase the risk of cancer. Another study published in the Journal of the National Cancer Institute [5] found women with elevated testosterone or decreased progesterone to be at increased risk of breast cancer.

However, when medroxyprogesterone was introduced to hormone replacement therapy, it did all that doctors and researchers believed was needed: it protected the uterus lining from overgrowth caused by estrogen given alone and reduced the risk of endometrial cancer. It seems that its effect on breast tissue was not part of the research done on this drug at that time.

In the early 2000's, doctors started to notice the results of studies[6] [7] indicating that the standard regimen of hormone replacement therapy was causing more harm than good overall, and many began recommending women stop taking these hormones right away, sometimes simply refusing to renew their prescriptions. Although, as mentioned earlier, later studies suggested more

---

[4] . Chang K, et al, Fertil Steril. 1995 Apr;63(4):785-91, Influences of percutaneous administration of estradiol and progesterone on human breast epithelial cell cycle in vivo.

[5] https://academic.oup.com/jnci/article/97/10/755/2544018

[6] . Women's Health Initiative Study (WHI), 1991-2002

[7] . Women's International Study of Long Duration Oestrogen after Menopause (WISDOM), 1999-2002

benefit and reduced risk in symptomatic women less than 60 years old, as compared to older women without symptoms,8 hormone supplement use for menopause symptoms dropped dramatically. While some women adjusted to the sudden stop of their hormone treatment without excessive difficulty, there were many who suffered terribly with the abrupt change in hormone levels this caused.

---

[8] . Salpeter S: Mortality associated with hormone replacement therapy in younger and older women. J Gen Intern Med. 2004,19:791-804.

CHAPTER THREE

WHAT IS A NORMAL CYCLE?

To more easily understand what changes at menopause, I find it helpful to thoroughly understand the normal cycle that occurs each month. Your body gives subtle signs that tell you what is happening in your hormone cycle. Learning to "read" these can help you achieve or avoid pregnancy, and know when, how and why your cycle changes.

The first day of menstrual bleeding was chosen as the beginning of the cycle for no specific reason. A woman's period is really the end result of what happened earlier in the cycle. However, for the purposes of this explanation, we will begin as usual, with the first day of menstruation, referred to as "day 1" of a woman's cycle.

Days of the cycle

When menstruation begins, both estrogens and progesterone are at the low point of production. Menstruation, itself, is the shedding of the lining of the uterus (called the endometrium) that was built up by hormone action earlier in the cycle. This shedding occurs because the levels of hormone have become too low to support growth and maintenance of this tissue. A normal menstrual flow can last 2 to 7 days and may vary from month to month and still be considered normal. Basically, a "normal" period is what is normal for you!

Chart (explained in text below):

BEGINNING OF CYCLE (at end of period)
Low E (estrogen) and P (progesterone) in the blood
↓
Sensed by hypothalamus (menstrual control center), signals pituitary
↓
Pituitary releases FSH (follicle stimulating hormone) into blood
↓
FSH stimulates follicles in ovary
↓
Follicles produce E
↓
One follicle becomes dominant (others shrink)
↓
Egg inside develops

OVULATION
Very high Estrogen in blood
↓
Sensed by hypothalamus, signals pituitary

↓

Pituitary releases a surge of LH (luteinizing hormone)

↓

Follicle ruptures, releasing egg

MENSTRUATION

Sac left behind on ovary = Corpus luteum

↓

Corpus luteum produces estrogen and progesterone

↓

E and P sensed by hypothalamus, signals pituitary

↓

Pituitary decreases production of FSH and LH

↓

E and P production by corpus luteum decreases

↓

Too low hormone to support endometrium, period starts

PREGNANCY

Fertilized egg begins secreting hCG (human chorionic gonadotropin) when it implants in uterus

↓

HCG supports corpus luteum to continue hormone production, maintains pregnancy until the placenta takes over

After the menstrual period, estrogen and progesterone in the blood are at low levels. The menstrual control center in the hypothalamus area of the brain "reads" the levels of hormone in the blood. When it senses low levels of reproductive hormones, it signals the pituitary to release Follicle Stimulating Hormone (FSH), and FSH travels through the blood, signals the ovaries, and triggers several follicles to begin to enlarge and secrete estrogen. This causes blood estrogen to begin to increase. Estrogen stimulates the endometrium causing the cells to grow and divide, thickening this lining of the uterus. At the same time, vaginal secretions, produced by glands in the endometrium, also respond to increased levels of estrogen, increasing in volume and becoming "eggwhite-like" in texture (clear, wet, and stretchy, with a lubricating quality, much like the white of an egg). Women will watch for the presence of this fluid, referred to as vaginal mucous, to indicate estrogen levels have increased and the ovulation cycle has begun.

Eventually, one follicle becomes dominant, while the others whither, and the egg (or "ovum") inside develops. Occasionally, more than one follicle will remain dominant and, if both eggs were released and fertilized, this would result in fraternal twins.

When estrogen reaches a high level, the pituitary releases a surge of another hormone, called Luteinizing Hormone (LH) that triggers the dominant follicle to rupture, releasing its egg. This is called ovulation. Once ovulation has occurred, estrogen production by the follicle drops somewhat then rises again a few days later. The empty follicle can be seen on the surface of the ovary as a tiny yellowish spot and is referred to as the "corpus luteum" which means "yellow body" in Latin.

The corpus luteum continues to produce estrogen, creating the second wave of this hormone, and it also begins to produce large amounts (in comparison to estrogen) of a second hormone, progesterone. The amounts of estrogen produced per day are measured in micrograms, while amounts of progesterone per day are measured in milligrams, units of measure that are 1000 times greater.

The name progesterone was derived from "pro-gestational hormone" as it is essential to establish and continue a pregnancy (or "gestation"). The day that ovulation occurs is sometimes referred to as the "peak" day, describing the peak of blood estrogen as well as the peak production of vaginal mucous.

Tracking your hormones

Women have used the presence of vaginal mucous to monitor their cycle for many years, determining their fertile days in order to either achieve or avoid pregnancy. The simplest method is to observe the amount of mucous present each day. Increasing amounts of mucous production signal that ovulation is approaching. At ovulation, the mucous changes from clear and "stretchy" (like an egg white in texture) to a creamy white or light yellow.

When applied to a glass slide, this mucous will dry in a pattern of beautiful ferns that form closer together as estrogen levels rise. This is referred to as "ferning" and has been used by physicians for many years as a simple way to ensure women who want to conceive are producing enough estrogen. As the ferning is barely visible to the naked eye, the slide must be magnified to monitor the changes in ferns as estrogen increases.

Ferning also changes with the cycle: estrogen in clear body fluids, such as saliva or vaginal mucous, follows the rising and falling of estrogen in the blood. The ferns of dried estrogen form more and more closely together as estrogen production increases. When progesterone is produced at ovulation, the ferns become blobby and noticeably less crisp. These changes allow the prediction and detection of ovulation. Tracking the menstrual cycle by daily observation of dried saliva or vaginal mucous on a glass slide with a small microscope is simple to do and far less expensive than using ovulation prediction kits that are available in drug stores. An inexpensive microscope can be purchased on the internet for this purpose. Usually saliva, which shows the same results as vaginal fluids, is used for convenience.

A guideline for those wishing to achieve (or avoid) pregnancy, is that both the presence of "eggwhite-like" mucous and the formation of ferns in dried mucous are indicative of fertile days in a normal cycle. Wet mucous is actually necessary to enable movement of sperm in the female reproductive tract and passage through the cervix. A lack of mucous is referred to as a "dry cycle" and can be a contributing cause of fertility problems.

If the egg or ovum is fertilized by a sperm, cell division begins and the zygote, as it is now called, continues through the fallopian tubes to the uterus where it implants into its thickened lining. The implanted fertilized ovum produces human Chorionic Gonadotropin or hCG (the hormone detected by pregnancy tests), which maintains the corpus luteum. With a fertilized ovum, the corpus luteum continues to produce progesterone for the next 12 weeks, sustaining the pregnancy until the placenta takes over the production of progesterone for the remainder of the pregnancy.

Progesterone and another lesser-known hormone called inhibin, produced at ovulation, travel through the blood stream and are detected by the menstrual control center in the hypothalamus of the brain. These hormones signal the hypothalamus to reduce its production of FSH and LH, the hormones that drive the ovaries to produce estrogen and the ovum (egg).

If the egg is not fertilized, it dissolves and, since no hCG is being produced, the corpus luteum shrinks and stops producing estrogen and progesterone. With the falling levels of these hormones we are back to day 1 of the cycle - the thickened lining of the uterus is no longer sustained and sheds, creating the vaginal drainage of tissue, fluids and blood that women know as menstruation.

You can readily see that this is a complex system with multiple areas where interference could disrupt the delicate balance of the normal cycle. In the following chapters, I will discuss some of the ways the cycle can become unbalanced or disrupted, and how we can work to normalize the cycle again.

If you are interested in learning more about monitoring your reproductive cycle, I recommend "Taking Charge of Your Fertility" by Toni Weschler as an excellent and very interesting resource.

CHAPTER FOUR

HOW DO HORMONES ACT IN THE BODY?

Estrogens

Estradiol, estrone and estriol are the 3 main estrogens, but there are over a dozen estrogens in the human body, some strong and some weak, and the balance between these is important. Stronger estrogens give us the hormone actions we need, while weaker ones appear to play a protective role.

Estrogens act on many tissues in the body, from our skin, blood clotting, bone and brain, to the uterus, vagina, breast and ovaries, and more. While estrogen is known for its ability to stimulate tissues that are involved in reproduction, such as growth of breast tissue and the endometrial lining of the uterus, it also generally stimulates growth of many other areas of the body. These are referred to as "estrogen-responsive" tissues. Overall, it is a hormone that encourages growth and activity of receptive body cells.

Progestogens

Progesterone is the main hormone in its class in the human body, known as progestogens. There is some confusion about the terms progestogen (also sometimes spelled "progestagen"), progestin and progesterone. Progestogen is the name of a group or "class" of hormones which have a particular action on the uterus; progesterone is the main human hormone in this class; and the term, progestin, refers to synthetic versions of progesterone that are not found naturally in the human body.

There are many synthetic progestins that are commercially available in addition to medroxyprogesterone that was discussed earlier. Many of these are used in birth control pills. Progestogens all prevent overgrowth of the endometrial lining of the uterus. However, our own progesterone acts on many other tissues in the body as well. These include stimulating growth in bone, reducing cell division in the breast, creating relaxant effects in the brain, reducing clotting in the blood and helping to create an anti-inflammatory effect through the immune system. Progesterone is necessary to support a pregnancy (or gestation) and the name "progesterone" is derived from this action: "Pro-gestational-hormone". Progesterone receptors have also been identified on the protective myelin sheath that insulates nerves (the tissue that is damaged in Multiple Sclerosis), suggesting the possibility of a protective action on nerve cells as well.

However, synthetic progestins, while keeping a progesterone-like effect on the uterus lining, may have different effects at these other sites that can vary between different progestins because of their differing structures. One notable difference is that progesterone is needed to support pregnancy while the synthetic version, medroxyprogesterone, must be avoided in pregnancy, indicating that this synthetic version of progesterone must actually block an essential action of the natural hormone at an important site during pregnancy.

Androgens

Testosterone is the main androgen used in hormone replacement for both men and women when needed. Testosterone is responsible for the development of characteristics considered to be masculine: facial and body hair growth, development of male sexual organs, growth of bone (including the brow ridge and jaw, giving male facial characteristics), deepening of the voice, etc. It is available commercially, but it is also manufactured as synthetic testosterone compounds, sometimes called "testosterone salts", that are well absorbed when taken by mouth but have a risk of causing liver damage with extended use. Manufacturers addressed this problem by introducing transdermal testosterone cream and patches, identical to the hormone our bodies make, in dosages appropriate for men's hormone replacement.

Although estrogen is the hormone class that gives a person female characteristics while testosterone produces male traits, men and women produce both of these hormones. It is the balance between the two that promotes the features that we use to define gender, but both sexes require both estrogen and testosterone in proper amounts to be healthy and balanced.

Women generally produce about one-tenth the amount of testosterone that men produce so, although doctors will sometimes prescribe a commercial testosterone supplement that was designed for men, it is easy for women to overdose when taking one of these.

Symptoms of overdose include acne, facial hair growth and, if taken at high enough dose for long enough, deepening of the voice. These symptoms gradually reverse when the hormone is discontinued, except for voice changes.

Thyroid

The thyroid is sometimes referred to as the "master gland" of the body, as its hormone is necessary for the function of every cell in the body. The thyroid gland is located at the base of the front of the neck and it produces two main thyroid hormones, T3 and T4 (also known as Liothyronine and Levothyroxine).

The numbers, 3 and 4, indicate how many iodine molecules are attached to the thyroid hormone. Much more T4 is produced than T3, but T3 is more active than T4. Once inside the cell, T4 is changed to T3 by an enzyme that removes one molecule of iodine, increasing its activity. Selenium also forms part of the iodine hormone molecule. So, low intake of either iodine or selenium can be a cause of low thyroid production. Autoimmune disease, or Hashimoto's Thyroiditis, where the body's immune system mistakenly attacks the thyroid gland, is a major cause of low thyroid.

Low thyroid level, known as hypothyroidism or goitre, is one of the more common forms of hormone imbalances. Because thyroid hormone affects all cells, the symptoms are widespread. They include low body temperature, fatigue, hair loss, constipation, weight gain, frequent headaches, irregular periods, mood swings (especially anxiety, panic or phobia), muscle aches and pains not related to exercise, skin problems (adult acne, eczema or severe dry skin), and others. Low thyroid can also be responsible for excessive menopause symptoms that are not well relieved by estrogen.

So, you can readily see that hypothyroidism, even slight, can contribute to many different seemingly unrelated health problems. It can be difficult to find a successful menopause treatment if your thyroid is not functioning properly.

Low thyroid is most easily diagnosed by blood tests. While levels of T4 and T3 can be measured in the blood, doctors usually measure another hormone, thyroid stimulating hormone (TSH), that is produced by the pituitary gland, located near the base of the brain. TSH is the hormone that stimulates the thyroid gland to make its hormones. When the brain detects that thyroid hormones are low, it signals the pituitary gland to produce more TSH to get the thyroid going. So, a high TSH means that your blood thyroid must be low. This test is also used to regulate the dose of thyroid when you are taking it. A high TSH signals your doctor to increase the dose. If TSH becomes too low, this tells your doctor that you are likely taking too much thyroid replacement.

However, there is a controversy around what a "normal" range of TSH is. A range of 0.5 to 5 was used for years, but this has been lowered to 0.5 to 4.5 and even 0.3 to 3.0 in some areas. Some doctors have observed that their patients feel their best when TSH is near 1. Since too much thyroid hormone puts a person at risk of developing osteoporosis, there is a tendency to under-dose with this hormone to reduce this risk. However, even slight under-dosing can leave the patient feeling less than their best.

The other factor in diagnosing and monitoring thyroid, is that T4 is converted into the more active T3 mostly inside our cells.

Blood tests can only detect what is in the blood. Some researchers have suggested that some individuals, particularly under the influence of extreme stress, may have difficulty converting T4 into T3 inside their cells, creating reverse-T3 (an inactive form of T3) instead. This has been named "Wilson's Thyroid Syndrome" after the doctor who first proposed this theory. While considered controversial, it could explain the extreme fatigue and hypothyroid-like symptoms some individuals experience after severe stress. While thyroid replacement is usually done using only T4 (Levothyroxine), these patients would benefit from converting part of the dose to T3 (Liothyronine) because of these conversion problems.

So, managing hypothyroidism can be complex. If you have several of the symptoms listed above, talk to your doctor about having a thyroid blood test at your next check-up. Meanwhile, you could take your temperature several times a day for a few days; a consistently low average body temperature suggests your thyroid may not be functioning optimally. This was the method of testing that was used by physicians before blood tests were developed. A continuing low body temperature with treatment, however, suggests that the dosage or type of thyroid hormone replacement is likely not optimal.

Note also that the thyroid can become overactive, called hyperthyroidism or Graves' disease. Overactivity can be caused by tumors, non-cancerous nodes, or thyroiditis (inflammation of the thyroid gland). Symptoms of excess thyroid hormone include excessive sweating, heat intolerance, increased bowel movements, tremor, nervousness, agitation, anxiety, increased heart rate or heart palpitations, weight loss, fatigue and weakness. It is treated by administering radioactive iodine to reduce thyroid function, by drugs that block thyroid, or by surgery. Often people will need to take thyroid supplements after treatment, particularly with radioactive iodine or surgery, as too little thyroid function may remain after the treatment.

Adrenal hormones

You have two adrenal glands that are located on top of each kidney. They produce several different types of hormones, including ones that control minerals, most importantly sodium, which controls fluid balance, blood volume and blood pressure in the body. Some blood pressure medications work by influencing the activity of these hormones. The adrenals also produce some androgens, mainly testosterone and DHEA (dehydroepiandrosterone). After menopause, this supply of hormones tends to become more important in women, providing an ongoing source of hormone as ovaries reduce production.

Your adrenal glands also produce stress hormones: cortisol and adrenalin. Adrenalin triggers changes in body functions that help to enable a quick response to an emergency, while cortisol is a longer-acting stress hormone that keeps you alert and ready to respond to stressful events. Adrenalin (also known as epinephrine) is the hormone in EpiPen that is used to treat an extreme form of allergic reaction, called anaphylaxis. These stress hormones increase heart rate, raise blood sugar, divert blood supply from digestion to muscle, and keep you more alert.

Throughout human evolution, these hormones have helped us fight off or run from danger. This is often called our "fight or flight" response. However, now most of our stress is not the kind we can readily run from or physically fight off. But our stress hormone system is still preparing us to do this. Continual ongoing stress can keep our cortisol elevated, contributing to high blood pressure, risk for diabetes, and increased blood cholesterol... all these together create a condition called "metabolic syndrome", that is known to contribute to increased risk of disease, particularly heart disease and stroke.

Stress hormones are structurally similar to our reproductive hormones, and all are created from cholesterol molecules, as you will see in the charts below. Because estrogen and stress hormones have a similar structure and shape, a stressful event can bring on a hot flash. Here's how it happens...

Like a lock and key...

Hormones act by interacting with hormone receptors. I often explain this action by using the analogy of a lock and key: the key fits into the lock and if it is the correct key, it will turn the lock and open the door; a hormone fits into a receptor on the surface of a cell and, if it is the right hormone, it will turn on the receptor, creating an action within the cell. Incorrect hormones can sometimes fit into a receptor, blocking out the proper hormone but not turning it on, just as incorrect keys can sometimes fit into a lock but not turn. Others may fit into a receptor and keep it turned on longer than normal.

Excess amounts of one hormone can also change the action of another, giving the effect of a lack of a similar hormone even if normal amounts of it are present. Researchers believe this occurs because of competition for binding at the receptors.

One example of this hormone competition is a surge in production of the stress hormone, cortisol, blocking the effect of estrogen and bringing on hot flashes when a person is nervous or stressed. Another example is excess production of estrogen with insufficient progesterone to balance, blocking the action of thyroid hormone and giving symptoms of low thyroid in spite of normal thyroid blood levels.

Environmental hormone-like chemicals can also fit into the receptor and either block it or stimulate it longer or more strongly than the natural hormone would. We sometimes refer to these estrogen-like environmental chemicals as "xenoestrogens" and they can have devastating effects when exposure occurs at critical times of human growth as I will discuss in the next chapter.

Reproductive hormones are rather large complicated molecules. They all contain a basic 4-ring structure, with changes in the side chains or bonding of the ring structure as the only differences. When I look at a chart of hormone production and metabolism in the body, I often think of the childhood game, "find the 2 drawings that are identical", because the chemical structures look so similar. The body can metabolize one hormone into another, following a series of changes that begin with a cholesterol molecule. I have always wondered if reducing cholesterol to an extremely low level in an attempt to prevent or treat heart disease might result in insufficient cholesterol to create the hormones we need. However, I have never seen any studies that have demonstrated this, although it could be because no one has looked.

The following is a diagram of hormone structures. Starting with cholesterol in the upper left, the arrows show the pathways of the creation of estrogen, progesterone, testosterone and adrenal gland hormones that control minerals, fluid and the stress response:

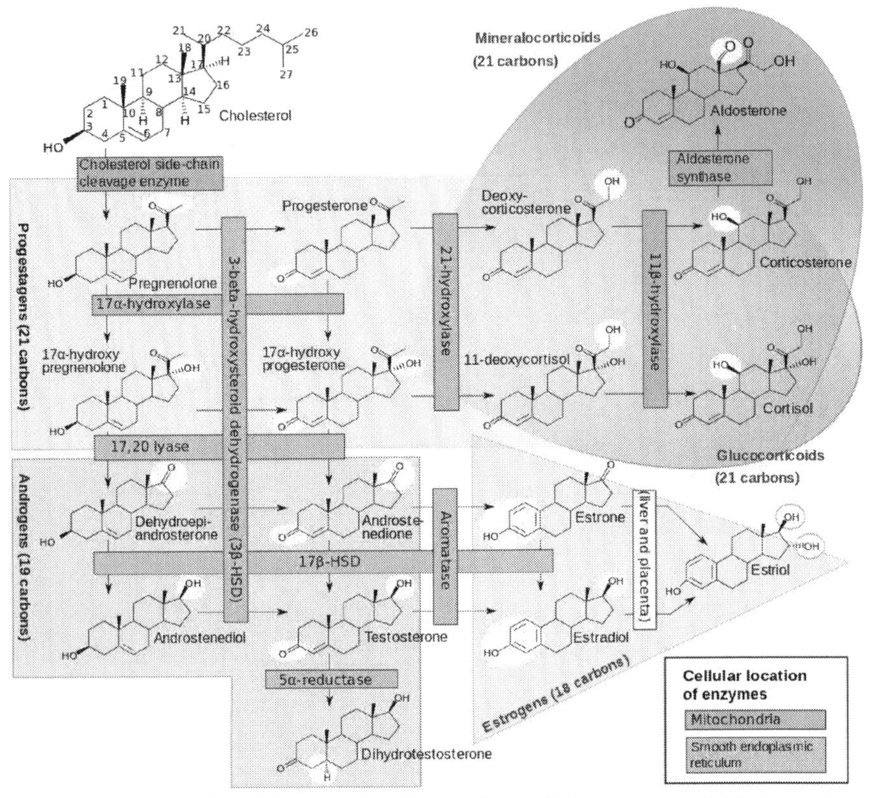

Human steroidogenesis, with the major classes of steroid hormones, individual steroids and enzymatic pathways. Changes in molecular structure from a precursor are highlighted in white.

Credit: Häggström M, Richfield D (2014). "Diagram of the pathways of human steroidogenesis".Wikiversity Journal of Medicine1(1).DOI:10.15347/wjm/2014.005.ISSN20018762.

In this chart, (if you are viewing the color version) color coding helps to show the different classes of hormone, with progestogens in yellow, androgens (including testosterone) in blue, and estrogens in pink. The purple area indicates the mineralocorticoids that control our minerals and fluid balance, and the green area shows cortisol, our main stress hormone. You can see that they all contain a similar 4-ring structure with variations in side changes being responsible for the changes in activity of the different hormones. The arrows show how one is metabolized into another, with the green and orange strips noting the enzyme that is needed for the modification. The chart below demonstrates one way that stress is believed to influence our hormone production, with the demand for extra production of stress hormones leading to reduced production of androgens and estrogens.

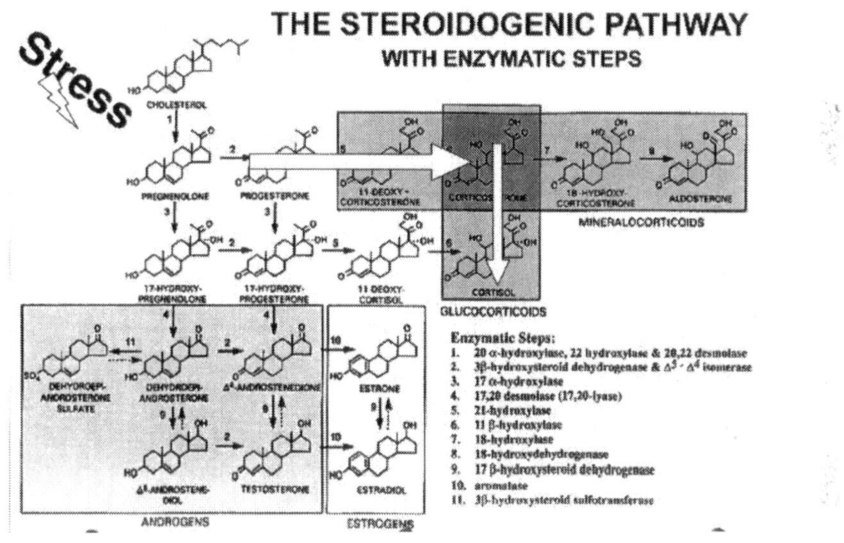

Credit: Professional Compounding Centres of America (PCCA) course materials

As mentioned in the discussion of progesterone versus medroxyprogesterone, different parts of these complex molecules act at different locations in the body: one section might fit in one type of receptor in the breast, while a different area of the hormone might fit into a different receptor in the uterus. With estrogens, three different types of receptors have been identified: ER-a (or estrogen receptor "a"), ER-b and ER-c, signifying 3 different active areas of estrogen molecules that fit into 3 different types of receptors. Some estrogens will have a weak or even a blocking effect on one receptor but will act more strongly on another. This has lead to the development of what some refer to as "designer estrogens", trying to maintain the beneficial effects of estrogen, such as protecting against bone loss and preventing hot flashes, while avoiding the negative effects of estrogen, such as overstimulation of the breast or uterus tissues that can lead to increased cancer risk.

Two designer estrogens on the market are tamoxifen and reloxifene. Tamoxifen is marketed for its protective effect on the breast but is known to be associated with an increased risk of endometrial cancer. Reloxifene is marketed for protection against bone loss but has also been found to decrease the risk of invasive breast cancer. It does not stimulate growth of the lining of the uterus. Both drugs cause increased hot flashes and increased risk of blood clots as a side effect.

While the ideal synthetic designer estrogen has not yet been marketed, our own weak estrogen, estriol, appears to be what they should be aiming for: it does not stimulate the endometrial lining of the uterus or the breast, it does not increase blood clotting, it greatly improves the vaginal lining and helps somewhat to improve hot flashes. The jury is still out, however, on whether it helps to protect bone, as some studies have found it helpful while others found its effect on bone to be neutral. Estriol, this natural protective estrogen that our bodies produce in high amounts especially during pregnancy, is very poorly absorbed by mouth, so has little effect in pill form. It would seem logical to me, however, to work on an alternative administration method to take advantage of its beneficial properties – perhaps a transdermal patch, cream or gel, or even a suppository – rather than trying to "recreate the wheel" with substitutes. I have often recommended it for women with vaginal atrophy or dryness, for whom non-medicated lubricant gels were insufficiently helpful, especially when they wanted minimal therapy. Results from this use appeared to be comparable to creams and suppositories containing stronger estrogens.

CHAPTER FIVE

ARE THERE HORMONES IN THE ENVIRONMENT?

A personal experience

When I was young, many chemicals were readily available for household use that have subsequently been banned or restricted due to harmful effects. My parents were avid gardeners and, although they handled these agents carefully and applied them according to directions, all of my family was exposed, probably more than average... especially my Dad. A beautiful lawn and a weed- and pest-free garden were easier to achieve when pesticides and herbicides were used. Names like malathion and 2,4-D were household terms in our home, along with DDT that was painted on the screens of our cottage porch where we ate most of our meals. I still remember the pesticide's smell, and how it stayed on your hands if you happened to touch one of the large screens. These chemicals were all considered quite safe to use at the time.

My father, of course, being the person who applied most of the chemicals, received the most exposure. On his 51st birthday, after a significant intentional loss of weight, he was diagnosed with acute leukemia, and he died from it about six months later.

Most of these hormone-disrupting chemicals, like the hormones normally produced by our bodies, are oil soluble and stored in fatty tissues. Rapid weight loss can flood the body with these stored chemicals, creating an acute exposure from within. Although never actually confirmed by doctors, this is what we believe happened to my father – it seemed the only reasonable explanation for an adult suddenly developing a disease that occurs most often in childhood. Researchers have determined that many small exposures to fat soluble substances over time can be a toxic equivalent to a single heavy exposure because these chemicals are stored in the body.9 Most weight loss experts now recommend a gradual weight loss to minimize the impact of released toxins, and drinking plenty of fluids during weight loss to ensure these toxins are flushed out of the body quickly. This experience made me aware of harmful, sometimes hormonally active, substances in the environment and piqued my interest to learn more.

Perimenopause has changed

I was much less exposed to these chemicals than my father, but I suspect it was enough to create problems with a hormone imbalance I experienced later. I was fascinated with literature describing the appearance of large numbers of women with

---

[9] . Documentary film: Exposure: Environmental Links to Breast Cancer, A Butterfield Zuckerman Production, 1997. Available at www.womenshealthyenviromnents.ca/films/ in English, (plus French and Spanish – VHS version only), along with 2009 60-page resource guide.

hormone imbalances, like mine, that weren't described in textbooks of earlier generations. Physicians, Dr. Jerilynn Prior10 and Dr. John Lee documented a different experience in their patients in the months and years leading to menopause than they had learned about in medical school.

Their textbooks described menopause as a slow decline of the ovaries, which stopped ovulating when they ran out of eggs. Most textbooks still describe menopause this way. However, in many women, ovulation stops months or years before menopause, while the ovaries are still capable of producing plenty of estrogen. When ovulation does not occur, progesterone is not released and the brain sends increasing amounts of signaling hormones, LH and FSH, to stimulate hormone production by the ovaries. These partially functioning ovaries can become overstimulated, producing much larger amounts of estrogen than normal but little or no progesterone. This is because it is the sac that is left behind after the ovulation that produces the majority of our progesterone... no egg production means no sac and no production of progesterone by the ovaries.

This scenario creates a dramatic hormone imbalance, with high estrogen and low progesterone. Dr. Prior's research describes about 40% of women in perimenopause with this imbalance but gynecology textbooks she studied, as a medical student, did not mention this phenomenon at all. Dr. Lee recorded his observations of patients with similar imbalances in his book "What Your Doctor May Not Tell You About Perimenopause".11

---

[10] . Prior JC,Perimenopause: The Ovary's Frustrating Grand Finale, BC Endocrine Research Foundation, Vol 3, No.3, Fall 2001.

[11] . Lee J, What Your Doctor May Not Tell You About Perimenopause, ISBN 0-446-67380-3, 1999

Timing of exposure is important

Hormone-disrupting chemicals are believed to have a greater effect when the exposure occurs during certain times of human development or growth. For example, diethylstilbestrol (DES), a hormone drug used from the 1940s until the late 1960s to prevent miscarriage, only had a noticeable detrimental effect on health when administered during pregnancy at a precise time in the development of the female fetus – the time that the ovaries and uterus were developing. This makes sense: a hormone-disrupting chemical (or synthetic hormone) would cause maximum damage when it is blocking a human hormone the developing organ needs for growth.

When given at just the wrong time, DES could cause malformations in the reproductive organs that were only detectable in women years later when her menstrual cycles began. These women could have extremely heavy menstrual flows and were eventually found to have a higher risk of cancers of the reproductive system. In male children, higher rates of malformations of the penis, called hypospadias, were noted.

Fortunately, studies demonstrated that DES was not effective in preventing miscarriages and its use declined even before it was known to cause birth defects. Use during pregnancy was officially banned in 1971, when a report was published describing a probable link between DES and a rare type of vaginal cancer, although it continued to be used for additional years for menopausal complaints, such as urinary incontinence (leaky bladder).

There was an active campaign for a number of years, looking for these "DES daughters" who were at higher risk of cancer – women whose mothers were given DES during pregnancy – to try to detect any resulting cancers at an early treatable stage.

An example from nature

An interesting study was published in 1997, about alligators living in Lane Apopka in Florida where a spill of pesticide had occurred.12 The spill was treated and the water was cleared of contaminants, but the alligators were not reproducing. An examination of their reproductive organs revealed that the males' penises were smaller than normal and the females' ovaries were described as being "burned out". The authors of the study stated that the animals had been "estrogenized", or exposed to an estrogen-like chemical. It was determined that, although the water was clear, the plants and smaller animals had taken up the pesticide. With the alligators at the top of the "food chain", the pesticide effect was concentrated and manifested in the form of reproductive problems.

So, this is an example of the effects of an acute exposure to these toxins, but what about a more subtle exposure?

A follow up to the study above compared alligators in Lake Apopka (which had a major chemical spill) plus those in Lake Okeechobee (which had numerous contaminant sources but no major spill), with alligators in a "control" lake, Lake Woodruff (which remained uncontaminated). The alligators in Lakes Apopka

[12] . Semenza JC, et al, Reproductive Toxins and Alligator Abnormalities in Lake Apopka Florida, Environ Health Perspect, 105:1030-1032 (1997).

and Okeechobee exhibited similar hormone related changes that were not seen in Lake Woodruff alligators.[13] This suggests that a low level exposure to hormone disrupting chemicals can have detrimental health effects similar to those of an acute exposure (depending on the level of exposure over time), and is likely due to the body's ability to store these fat-soluble substances in our body fat.

One difficulty in linking the effect of hormone disrupting substances with health problems is the lag time in detecting these problems. Researchers may need to look back many years to find the cause and must consider the possibility of other contributing factors since that time. Unfortunately, the cost of environmental research and competition for available research dollars limit the amount of investigation into these issues.

Humans, like alligators, are at the top of the "food chain"- it is logical that some of our reproductive problems (such as decreased fertility) may be from concentration and storage of lower amounts of environmental chemicals over a period of many years. This process could also be the background cause of higher rates of menopausal problems we see in some cultures.

In humans, with much lower exposure than what those alligators would have experienced, the results would be expected to be much more subtle. Rather than "burned out" ovaries as found in the alligator study, low exposure over a period of time could result in seemingly normal ovaries that do not continue to function fully for the expected number of years. This could explain the

---

[13] . Grain DA, et al, Sex-steroid and thyroid hormone concentrations in juvenile alligators (Alligator mississippiensis) from contaminated and reference lakes in Florida, USA. Environmental Toxicology and Chemistry, 1998.

perimenopausal ovary dysfunction described by Dr. Prior and Dr. Lee.

More on the environment

A close friend of mine was diagnosed with an aggressive breast cancer when we were both 41. Fortunately, it was caught early and successfully treated. We are both in our 60s now, and she is healthy with no sign of the return of the cancer. I mention this because she took me to a lecture about environmental connections to breast cancer not long after her treatments were finished. It was an eye-opener for everyone in the room. The documentary film, Exposure, was presented by its producer and director.14 It was a 55-minute summary of research into environmental factors connected to increased rates of breast cancer, and they answered questions and continued the discussion afterward.

When we talk about a contaminated environment, most of us think of manufacturing plants polluting the air or water, or contamination drifting down wind from a nuclear plant. We think of toxins in the environment that can create hormone disruptions in our bodies. While these are important issues exposed in the documentary, the film also discussed the environment you create in your home, which is at least as important and much easier to control.

[14] . Documentary film: Exposure: Environmental Links to Breast Cancer, A Butterfield Zuckerman Production, 1997. Available at www.womenshealthyenviromnents.ca/films/ in English, (plus French and Spanish – VHS version only), along with 2009 60-page resource guide.

Chemicals, such as insecticides, break down more quickly outdoors in the sunshine and weather than they do inside the home. These chemicals should be used sparingly indoors, if at all. But, in addition to introducing potentially hormone-disrupting chemicals into the home, many of us unknowingly expose ourselves daily to other hormone disruptors. Hormone disruptors, like hormones, are generally fat-soluble substances, and the body readily stores these in its fatty tissues too. The documentary video "Exposure" discussed the many ways that hormone-blocking substances can enter the body and cause havoc and the discussion afterward suggested methods to avoid this exposure.

The chemicals my father used on the lawn and garden were thought to be safe when used as directed on the package label and, being a pharmacist, he followed the directions carefully, wearing a mask and protective clothing, and showering immediately afterward. These exposures were not immediately toxic but, because the chemicals accumulated in the fat stores in his body and were released later over a short time frame due to rapid weight loss, the effect was increased.

Observations in my clients caused me to suspect mild environmental hormone (xenohormone) exposures as a cause of hormone imbalance. Some women described playing in fog produced by insecticide-spraying trucks when children. These same women also complained of heavy flooding periods in the years before menopause that we associate with partial ovarian failure. Estrogen-like chemicals in the environment are also suspected of increasing risk of reproductive cancers (of the breast and uterus), particularly when the exposure is during a critical period of development such as before birth or during puberty. More research needs to be done in this area.

Plastic can have a hormonal effect

A woman who worked in a nearby store came into my pharmacy asking to talk to me about her hormone related problems. I noticed that she was holding a styrofoam plastic coffee cup, so I asked her if she drank her coffee in that type of cup very often. "Oh yes, every day... I like styrofoam cups with a plastic lid, because they keep my coffee hot!". Many plastics contain hormone-like chemicals and contact with food and drinks should be avoided to prevent ingestion and potential hormonal effects.

Styrofoam cups are essentially plastic foam and should never be used for hot drinks. Have you noticed a different taste when coffee is served in these? Look closely at the package... usually these are now labeled as cold drink cups. Unfortunately, some airlines and take-out restaurants continue to use them in spite of the danger being well established. Many travel coffee mugs, even some that appear to be stainless steel, are lined with plastic. Look inside before you buy if you plan to use these for hot drinks.

Microwaving food in plastic containers or covered with plastic wrap is another example of how potentially harmful hormone blocking substances can be introduced into the body through our food. Heat and direct contact with fatty food can result in increased transfer of plasticers, the substances that give plastic its flexibility, into your food. The softer the plastic, the more potential for harm, and it is almost impossible to know if a particular type of plastic has been completely tested for long-term safety. However, a numbering system is used to indicate types of plastic. Look for a number 1 to 7 printed inside a triangle on the plastic product:

numbers 2, 4 and 5 are considered most safe. Use numbers 1 and 7 with caution and avoid using numbers 3 and 6 for foods or drinks.

In addition to a hormone mimicking or hormone blocking effect in the body, these chemicals can also change the way your body breaks down hormones by altering liver function. It is recommended that you always microwave food in safe ceramic or glass dishes and cover with a glass lid, or at least ensure that any plastic lid does not touch the food to reduce the chance of ingesting harmful chemicals. Note that cling wrap is a number 3 plastic - if you must use it, prevent it from touching hot or fatty food.

It's also difficult to know what chemicals have been used to treat our food, whether from plant or animal sources. While governments regulate substances that can be used in food production, some of the older agents still being used were not evaluated by current standards. A series published in the Globe and Mail a few years ago described the massive task of re-examining the large number of chemicals currently in use, a job that will require years to complete. When you consider the difficulty in associating cause and effect when harm take years to detect, it makes sense to buy organic to reduce exposure to these chemicals as much as possible.

Controlling the environment within the home, where chemical exposure can be more concentrated, is something all of us can and should be doing. Sharing your concerns about potential hazards in the external environment with government authorities can also make a difference - many people voicing similar concerns can encourage regulators to act.

CHAPTER SIX

SHOULD I TAKE PILLS OR USE PATCHES?

When any medicine is swallowed, it must first dissolve in the stomach and/or intestines to enable the active ingredients to pass through membranes of the stomach and into the many blood vessels that surround your digestive system. Essentially all of these absorbed substances are then taken directly to the liver to be processed. This is referred to as the "first pass" through the liver where many drugs are broken down or removed from the bloodstream before they can reach rest of the body to act.

The liver is considered to be a type of filter... somewhat like a water treatment plant for the body. It eventually filters everything that enters our bodies, whether swallowed, inhaled or absorbed through the skin. It removes toxins, waste products and any substance our bodies detect as unfavorable. However, when drugs enter the body through the skin, they are circulated around the body before reaching the liver, avoiding the "first pass" effect, usually resulting in a lower dose being needed.

The liver removes some swallowed drugs more efficiently than others, and hormone supplements are very effectively removed. Because of this, doses of hormones given by mouth generally need to be significantly higher than when they are given by injection or transdermally (through the skin as a patch or penetrating cream). An exception to this rule is a hormone-like drug that is sufficiently different from our own hormones to avoid detection and processing by the enzyme systems in the liver. An example of this is medroxyprogesterone, as described earlier: the addition of the "medroxy" group to progesterone results in much less metabolism on the first pass through the liver.

An example of the difference in dosing with different routes of administration is the estrogen, estradiol. A common dose by mouth is 1 milligram (mg), equal to 1000 micrograms (mcg), that is taken once daily as a tablet. However, the same estradiol is used in transdermal patch form as doses of 25 to 50mcg, a far smaller amount at 1/20th of the oral dose.

Another example is progesterone. Literature describes it as "very poorly absorbed by mouth", but this isn't quite accurate. Progesterone is absorbed well enough but, as soon as it's absorbed, it goes directly to the liver where it is efficiently broken down before it reaches the rest of the body. Oral doses of progesterone are 100 to 300mg daily, but when administered as a transdermal cream, normal doses are 20 to 30mg daily. However, the extra 80 to 90% of progesterone that is needed when taken by mouth doesn't just disappear. It is metabolized into breakdown products that connect with "benzodiazepine" receptors in the brain.

Benzodiazepines are a class of drugs used as tranquillizers and sleeping pills - some examples are diazepam (Valium), alprazolam

(Xanax) and triazolam (Halcion). So, you can easily understand why a major side effect of oral progesterone is drowsiness! Note that progesterone cream, with its much lower dosing and fewer breakdown products, rarely causes any drowsiness.

So, what happens to the oral estrogen that the liver is filtering? The liver chemically changes much of it into other forms, some strong and some weak, which act on body receptors. A large percentage of the bioidentical hormone, estradiol, is changed when swallowed to the less favourable estrogen, estrone, that our bodies store and can release later. This is considered a negative factor as sometimes estrogen action is provided at a time when it is not wanted. This is seen in blood tests as increased levels of estrone even though the supplement given was estradiol. Some estrogens are excreted into the bowel for elimination via the gall bladder but can be reabsorbed into the system again if bowel conditions are favorable.

In addition, an increased amount of Sex Hormone Binding Globulin (SHBG), a protein that binds to estrogen and other hormones, is produced by the liver in response to estrogen that is swallowed. Hormone that becomes attached to the SHBG protein becomes inactive. So you can understand from all of these mechanisms why you need much higher amounts of hormone when you take it by mouth rather than transdermally or by injection.

Oral estrogens are also associated with gall bladder disease and androgens given by mouth are linked to liver cancers, presumably a result of the extra stress on the liver. As well, the dose of transdermal hormones is generally easier to adjust and women (and men!) should always strive to use the lowest effective dose of hormone. Most patches now have the hormone imbedded directly into the adhesive, rather than in a "puddle" or reservoir in the middle of the patch, and these types can be cut if necessary, without changing the absorption characteristics dramatically (whereas the reservoir type would release the pool of drug when cut). This allows for some ability to adjust the dose. When I compounded hormone creams, I generally preloaded them into syringes (without a needle, of course) so the client could simply squeeze out an accurate measure of the amount needed, and easily adjust the dose when necessary.

Because of these factors: reduced dose resulting in less side effects and less stress on the liver, plus easier adjustments and fine tuning of the dose, I generally favour the use of transdermal hormones rather than oral tablets or capsules.

But the liver does more with estrogen than described so far. We have over a dozen naturally produced estrogens in our bodies, many manufactured in the liver.

Think of the liver as a bag of enzymes – it is these enzymes that break down our hormones as well as many of the medications we take. Nutrients in our diet and chemicals introduced into our bodies, however, can influence which enzymes are more active.

Although our estrogen metabolism is very complex, I'll try to simplify it. There are two main enzyme systems we know about that metabolize estrogens: one system produces 2-hydroxy-estrone, a favourable form that is further changed into our weak protective estriol, and the other produces 16-alpha-hydroxy-estrone, a strong and less favourable estrogen. The balance between the good metabolism and the bad is believed by some experts to be a factor in the development of estrogen-related cancers. This can be measured as the ratio of 2- to 16-alpha hydroxyestrone in the blood.

Some foods, such as cruciferous vegetables, contain compounds that stimulate enzymes in the favourable system. This provides one possible explanation for the influence of diet on cancer risk.

Some environmental chemicals activate enzymes in the unfavourable system, explaining the identified link between environmental pollution and cancer. These chemicals are found in some pesticides, herbicides and plastics.

In my work with clients and presenting to women's groups, I have realized that many are not aware they can reduce your risk of exposure to harmful chemicals by avoiding contact between food and plastic and avoiding use of harmful chemicals in the home.

CHAPTER SEVEN

HOW TO ASSESS YOUR HORMONES

It is a challenge for your doctor to find time to analyze all of your symptoms during an appointment, especially with complex hormonal imbalances. However, if you prepare beforehand you will be ready to inform him/her exactly what needs to be addressed, even with minimum available time. This is what I did for clients – I helped them prepare for their appointment. I want to teach you to do this too.

I also went a step further, preparing a written summary of the client's main complaints – the symptoms she really needed fixed – and included suggestions, both prescription and non-prescription, for how these could be addressed. I learned that this process worked best when I delivered the report a few days before her appointment, allowing the doctor time to read and digest what I was saying. You may want to consider doing this as well to communicate more clearly and effectively.

While creating a written report may seem difficult for you to do as a patient, I can walk you through the process. You want to prepare yourself and your doctor ahead of time so the discussion you have during your appointment will communicate the severity of your situation and include your preferences for treatment. If your doctor is not familiar with the therapy you feel most comfortable with, he or she may not be prepared to prescribe it. Sometimes a doctor will say "no" simply because he doesn't know what to write on the prescription.

Be prepared to suggest returning at a later appointment, allowing him time to research your ideas and preferences. You could also offer to provide background prescribing information about your preferred therapy (included in this book). Remember, it is your body and you have a right to be included in the decision of what medications, if any, you will take. Your doctor is there to make sure your treatment is safe and effective. To make this easier for you, I have included additional documents I actually used with physicians in the Appendix at the end of this book.

With the information provided and some organization, you can write a "report" yourself. In this chapter, I will explain the thought process I used to gather the information I needed to communicate with women's physicians on their behalf. Use this process to analyze your symptoms as you read through this chapter. Make notes on the worksheet provided below (also in Appendix III) or simply on a sheet of paper. I have suggested a simple report format you can use to organize your information into a brief, concise written summary for your doctor at the end of this chapter.

Keep in mind that doctors are taught in medical school to prescribe only treatments that are "evidence based". This term means that there have been studies done with the treatment in question to show that it works and is safe to use. Since bioidentical hormones are not marketed commercially in Canada and only a few are available in US (mostly in health food stores), doctors are often not aware of the studies that have been done with this type of therapy. The saliva hormone testing company, ZRT Laboratory, has a page on its website www.salivatest.com, noted as "references", that documents a long list of referenced articles for patients and health professionals that few doctors have seen. I found many other hormone studies by searching Google Scholar, the version of Google that scans research literature, and learned about other studies by attending conferences, reading compounding journals and participating in online compounding discussion groups. I have included references to some of the most significant studies in this book. If your doctor is hesitant to prescribe the therapy you are interested in, providing studies or referenced documentation is the ideal way to communicate the validity of your choice. I have included samples of the documents I used to inform physicians in the Appendix.

This is the worksheet that I used for many years (also in Appendix III):

HORMONE CONSULT　　　　Payment discussed____

Date________________________　　　　Birthdate______________

Name__________________________　　　　Doctor________________

Phone_______________________________　　　　Email_________________

Address____

Current medications / Past Hormone-Related Medical History __________

____

____

Regular periods? ________________
Length______________________________
Frequency_________________________
Description____
____
Other cyclic symptoms
____
____

Pregnancies__________
Miscarriages_____________________
Difficulty in getting pregnant? ______
Surgeries_________________________

Main Concerns _______________
____
____

SYMPTOMS
Hot flashes____
Night sweats____
Vaginal dryness/mucous____
Urinary symptoms____
Insomnia____
Fluid retention____
Breast soreness____
Weight gain____
Headaches ____
Heart palpitations____
Memory change____
Moods____
Fatigue____
Hair loss/growth/skin changes____
Decreased muscle mass/strength______________________________________
Low libido____
Bone loss____
Joint pains/arthritis____
Bowel function____
Body temp____
Stress____

GOALS AND ASSESSMENT
____
____

It's a good idea to add your name and contact information to any written material you provide to your doctor – they receive volumes of paper daily, and you want this information to be added to your file. If you wish, you can print off the worksheet and make notes on your own symptoms as you read through the explanation below, or simply use a blank sheet of paper to note your significant symptoms and what they indicate.

Medications – Although your doctor should have a record of all the previous medications you have tried, it doesn't hurt to list them again with the results you have experienced. Include hormone related therapies that have been tried but failed. These are particularly informative for physicians. You want to make it as easy as possible for your doctor to understand why you are asking for a particular therapy, and failure of previous treatments is certainly a reason to consider an alternative, if that is what you are interested in.

Regular periods? Length, Frequency, Description – A detailed description of your menstrual cycle, next, can provide a lot of information: what the flow is like (how long; how heavy; whether it contains clots; whether it starts, stops then restarts early in the period; and what color it is at the beginning). A menstrual period that is brown or black at the very beginning rather than pink or red, stops then restarts, is very heavy, and contains blood clots suggests inadequate production of progesterone in proportion to estrogen production. This is described "estrogen dominance" because the action of estrogen dominates when there is not enough progesterone, the hormone that balances and opposes the action of estrogen.

If the period is extremely heavy and proceeded by severe fluid retention and breast soreness, this suggests that your estrogen level is also higher than normal, and that you may require a higher dose of progesterone, at least at the beginning of treatment, to balance the increased amount of estrogen that is being produced. Your doctor would be familiar with this concept as this is similar to the increased dose of synthetic progestin that is always required when women are prescribed a higher dose of administered estrogen. In the case study on a typical woman in perimenopause (in a later chapter), I describe how to know when you have enough progesterone to balance the amount of estrogen you are producing.

The discussion around reproductive history is to determine the possibility of a long-standing hormone imbalance. Difficulty in getting pregnant or problems in carrying a pregnancy to term could suggest a hormone problem may have existed years earlier, with difficulty producing sufficient progesterone. Progesterone, the "progestational hormone", as you will recall from Chapter 5, is necessary to establish and maintain pregnancy. It is always worthwhile to bring a long-standing hormone imbalance to your doctor's attention.

From this information, your doctor would likely already be starting to form an idea of what hormones you are producing and missing, but you want your him or her to have a complete picture of how you are feeling.

Main concerns – List the symptoms that most bother you, the ones you most need to have improved; concisely describe how these symptoms negatively affect your quality of life. For example, if you have bothersome night sweats, tell your doctor how often they wake you at night and whether this sleep disruption affects you during the day. Make notes to ensure that your descriptions will be brief but powerful, truly communicating the degree of disruption your symptoms are causing.

Symptoms – The list of symptoms on my worksheet is designed to check for various changes, some major and some minor, that would give clues to what hormones are missing or being overproduced. Rather than just a "yes or no" answer to whether a symptom occurs, information about how it has changed can be important as well. Consider each item on the list, read the description below of what I look for when meeting with clients and how I might interpret these details to form an overall picture of hormone production. Use this information to clearly describe your hormone related symptoms to your doctor.

Hot flashes, Night sweats – The list of specific symptoms on my worksheet starts with hot flashes and night sweats (which are really just a hot flash that occurs at night). Note how often they occur during the day ("hot flashes") and at night ("night sweats"), what makes them worse, and how much impact they have on your life. Many doctors, being male or too young, may not realize the degree to which a woman's life can be affected by the negative symptoms of the menopausal change. You want to communicate how devastating these symptoms are for you, clearly describing their frequency and severity.

Vaginal dryness/mucous – Vaginal symptoms, both dryness and its opposite -- excess mucous production -- provide information on hormone status. Dryness is usually believed to indicate too little estrogen being produced, but many health professionals don't realize that dryness can also be the result of low testosterone. Keep this in mind as some of our other symptoms are being considered: vaginal dryness can indicate low estrogen, low testosterone or both.

Vaginal "wetness", or the production of more vaginal mucous than normal, can result from high estrogen levels without sufficient progesterone to balance the estrogen. As you may recall from my description of a normal cycle in an earlier chapter, the production of vaginal mucous increases during the first week after a woman's period, coinciding with the increase in production of estrogen. So, it makes sense that this symptom can be used to determine approximately how high a woman's estrogen might be, whenever progesterone is not present. Vaginal secretions can also be used to determine the dose of progesterone that a woman needs: start with a low dose and gradually increase the daily amount until the vaginal mucous dries up or changes to a yellow or white creamy consistency.

The presence of clear, "slippery", lubricative mucous indicates plenty of estrogen is being produced but little or no progesterone; the greater the amount present, the higher the estrogen level is likely to be. Some women describe needing to wear a mini-pad to absorb the wetness caused by production of large amounts of clear vaginal mucous. Although it is normal to produce this type of mucous with increased estrogen production just before ovulation, the volume produced normally decreases with age. A large amount noted in a woman in mid-life suggests estrogen dominance, or "hyperstimulated ovary syndrome" with very high estrogen and non-existent progesterone, as described in writings by physician researcher, Dr. Jerilyn Prior and others. This syndrome is described in more detail in the case study on a typical perimenopausal client.

Urinary symptoms – Urinary symptoms, for example leakage during stresses such as sneezing or running, or outright incontinence, can indicate deterioration in genital tissues, in particular the urinary sphincter (the muscle that holds urine in), generally due to low estrogen production. Some women have decided to take hormones solely because of this distressing symptom. However, in some cases, urinary leakage can be corrected or at least improved by targeted exercises that increase muscle strength in the pubic area. Some physiotherapists offer training sessions that may eliminate the need for medication or can at least add to the effectiveness of a medical therapy. Be sure to discuss this option with your doctor before committing to any drug therapy.

Insomnia – Insomnia can be caused by hot flashes that occur during the night, but it can also be an independent symptom. Stress hormones, sometimes called "fight or flight" hormones, are designed to keep us alert, ready to fight off a danger or run from it. Of course, in cave man days such stress helped some people live through the night because it caused them to sleep lightly enough to wake quickly when a wild animal, that they knew was lurking in the neighbourhood, decided to attack.

Modern day stresses, however, like demanding jobs or unbalanced home/work schedules, can mean unrelenting stress that stimulates ongoing stress hormone production. Since these stress hormones keep you awake, a spurt of production during the night can be a cause of insomnia. Women, or men, who wake up at night for no reason and cannot return to sleep because "their mind is racing" may have produced a spike of stress hormones.

In addition to addressing the underlying stress problem (or your reaction to it), you could try taking pantothenic acid (vitamin B5) at bedtime. It can sometimes prevent this inappropriate stress hormone production. Try a dose of vitamin B5 at bedtime, or simply take a B-Complex vitamin that contains pantothenic acid. This offers a better option than taking sleeping pills that can be habit-forming.

The hormone, melatonin, is also used successfully by some to improve sleep. Melatonin is normally produced at bedtime, and its production is inhibited by light. Shift workers, who often need to sleep during the day, and those who have travelled through several time zones, sometimes do not produce their own melatonin temporarily. The body produces about 3mg daily, so it does not make sense to take more than would normally be produced. Melatonin is likely to work best in a person who is not producing their own normally. Like other hormones, swallowing results in a reduced dose reaching the system - as much as 2/3 of the swallowed dose - so it is best taken "sublingually" (dissolving the tablet under the tongue). Doses as low as 1/4 of a 3mg tablet have been found helpful, depending on the person's own production. Tablets of 5 and 10mg really don't make sense and should not be used. Hormones generally work best within a "normal" range... both higher and lower doses can have negative effects.

More ideas for non-medical treatment of sleeping problems, and programs that are available to help you, can be accessed at a Nova Scotia government sponsored site: www.sleepwellNS.ca .

Be very wary of prescription sleeping medications. Almost without exception these are designed for very short-term use (7-10 days) as they can be quite addicting. Rebound insomnia - increased difficulty sleeping for several days - often occurs when the medication is stopped, making it very difficult and uncomfortable to discontinue the medication.

Fluid retention, Breast soreness, Weight gain – Fluid retention, breast soreness and weight gain (especially around the hips and thighs) tend to occur together and indicate the presence of estrogen without progesterone. The worse they are, especially fluid retention and breast soreness, generally the higher the estrogen is likely to be.

Breast cells respond to the presence of estrogen by growing and dividing. If sufficient progesterone is also present, however, breast cell growth is prevented. The higher the level of estrogen that is present without progesterone, the more active the cell growth will be, and this is noted by how severe breast sensitivity, soreness and swelling becomes. Similarly, the greater the soreness/sensitivity, the higher the estrogen level is likely to be. Estrogen, again without progesterone present, creates a tendency to gain weight, especially around the hips and thighs.

While the descriptions of the period and vaginal fluids have already given clues about your estrogen and progesterone production, more symptoms mean stronger confirmation of an imbalance. Describing additional supporting symptoms can also help convince your doctor that you need some type of treatment to ease your suffering.

Headaches – Headaches can also be a symptom of hormone imbalance, but generally only when they occur in a pattern that coincides with the menstrual cycle. A lack of progesterone has been associated with some headaches and replacement has been found to be helpful in a few studies. It may be worth trying, especially if other supporting symptoms of low progesterone are present, and it's of interest to track whether headaches improve while treating other symptoms of low progesterone. However, this symptom alone would rarely be reason to prescribe hormone replacement.

Heart palpitations – Heart palpitations, or a sudden racing heartbeat, can also be a caused by high unbalanced estrogen, although many may not be aware of this. Of course, heart palpitations would be a reason to see your doctor to ensure it wasn't a serious condition. I have had clients, however, who were relieved to finally learn the probable cause of their heart palpitations was a hormone imbalance after having undergone extensive heart testing that revealed no problems.

When the symptom pattern suggests high, unbalanced estrogen, I also ask about "formication" or a strange sensation that feels like insects crawling on the skin. The name comes from "fourmis" which means "ant" in French. Women are often relieved, as with the heart palpitation described above, that it is merely due to their hormone imbalance and not something more serious or, worse, something they are simply imagining.

Memory Change, Moods – There are many receptors for estrogen, progesterone and testosterone in the brain, and irritability, anxiety and forgetfulness are common complaints when hormones are lacking or out of balance. Progesterone, in particular, has a calming, anti-anxiety effect. Also, some women note that their short-term memory improves after starting supplementation, especially for names and words that "just won't pop into their head" during conversation. Although I have never seen this symptom described in the scientific literature as associated with low progesterone, my observations with many women suggests that it likely is.

It appears that these receptors in the brain are specific for progesterone, and do not respond to synthetic alternative progestins. A pharmacist once described to me how embarrassing it was to be talking to another health professional and unable to remember the name of a drug she was very familiar with, and how this completely reversed after switching from medroxyprogesterone to progesterone.

Fatigue, Hair loss/growth, Decreased muscle mass/strength, Low libido – Fatigue can be caused simply by a lack of sleep due to waking caused by night sweats. However, low testosterone can also leave you feeling tired for no reason. As well, low testosterone is associated with a lack of interest, not only in sexual activity, but also in doing activities that you usually enjoy. Muscle mass and strength may be diminished, and low testosterone can leave you lacking in "a sense of wellbeing". Additionally, low testosterone can increase the risk of bone loss in both women and men.

One obvious symptom of low testosterone that I always ask about is decreased hair growth, notably in the pubic and axial (underarm) areas. Often women will also tell me that they only need to shave their legs occasionally or not at all, as compared to needing to shave every day or two when they were younger (when they would have had normal testosterone).

Replacing testosterone solely because of low libido (lack of interest in sex) is somewhat controversial, with studies that support using it and others that do not. Of course, low libido can be due to emotional or psychological factors, such as stress or relationship problems with one's partner. If you have supporting symptoms (such as body hair growth) or a blood or saliva test showing low testosterone, along with confirmation of a healthy, happy relationship, this is very helpful in confirming that the problem could be due to a lack of hormone.

It is important to ensure that women are not overdosed. However, we will often initially use an amount that is somewhat higher than normal production to replenish levels more quickly, if testosterone is very low. As mentioned earlier, women produce less than 1mg of testosterone daily; using a product designed for men generally provides 25 to 50mg per dose and creates a risk of causing significant side effects when used in women. I generally suggest using 2mg daily, transdermally (as a cream), for 2 weeks then reducing to 1mg or less daily. You want to try to determine your lowest effective dose - doses as low as 0.3mg daily have been found to be effective.15

Skin changes - Increased oiliness of the skin, especially along with increased acne skin eruptions, can indicate increased testosterone production (often due to cysts on the ovaries). Puberty begins with a surge of testosterone in both men and women and is a common cause of teenage acne. After menopause, the ovaries stop ovulating, resulting in a greatly reduced production of estrogen and progesterone. They do continue to produce androgens, however, which the body can convert into estrogens. The result of this pathway of hormone production, is a greater percentage of male-type hormone that manifests as a tendency toward acne blemishes for some women.

---

[15] S.Rako, The Hormone of Desire

Conversely, some skin changes are associated with low hormone levels. As we age, and our hormone levels naturally decline, we tend to have dryer skin with less oil production and need to pay more attention to skin care and moisturizing. Many years ago, estrogen was added to some skin creams for its benefit on the skin, but of course this is no longer accepted as we know estrogen is easily absorbed through the skin.

Bone loss - Bone density has been used as a measurement of bone health for many years, but the density of bone is only one parameter of bone health. The other component is bone strength which is much more difficult to measure. Information about the amount of weight-bearing exercise you have done over your lifetime, along with the results of a bone density test, can help assess your probability of sustaining a bone fracture in the future. The FRAX assessment (Fracture Risk Assessment Tool) also accounts for other risk factors for bone fracture. It is individualized for various countries and can easily be found by searching "FRAX" plus your country name on the internet.

Estrogen is well known to have a positive influence on bone density, but progesterone has also been shown to be involved in bone metabolism. In 1990, Canadian researcher, J Prior, demonstrated bone loss in young high-level women athletes who had stopped menstruating. (Prior, JC; N Engl J Med. 1990 Nov 1;323(18):1221-7)

Joint pains/arthritis - Progesterone is believed to have an anti-inflammatory effect and, as such, may exert a positive effect on mild joint inflammations. Mild joint pains or transient arthritis-like symptoms could be considered a secondary supportive symptom for low progesterone.

Bowel function, Body temperature – An important path of eliminating hormones from the body is via the bowels after being metabolized into more complex forms by the liver. Slow passage of bowel contents provides more time for bacteria in the bowel to break apart these complexes, allowing the hormones to be reabsorbed into the system. So, treating chronic constipation can create an improved hormone metabolism.

Chronic constipation can also by a symptom of low thyroid, along with low body temperature and low blood pressure, especially pressure that drops when moving from sitting to a standing position. Because it is more difficult to balance hormones when thyroid is lacking, I ask about these symptoms as well and bring them to the doctor's attention to encourage testing. On occasion, I would have a woman take her temperature several times a day, for a few days. A consistently low body temperature throughout the day also suggests low thyroid function.

Stress – Lastly, I always ask about stress. When humans are under chronic stress, we produce increased amounts of the stress hormone, cortisol. If you look back to the hormone metabolism chart in chapter 4, you will see that progesterone can be metabolized into cortisol, or into androgens or estrogens. If the demand for cortisol is increased, it is easy to see from this chart that a reduced production of androgens and estrogens could be the result. As well, being structurally similar to other hormones, excessive production of cortisol can block the action of androgens and estrogens, giving the effect of a drop in hormone level that has not actually occurred.

Goals and Assessment – Don't hesitate to tell your doctor what you think is going on and what your preferences for treatment are. Your appointment should be a conversation! Most of the time, there are several options you can try and your doctor should take your preferences into consideration. Studies have actually shown that patients are more likely to use a therapy if they have had input into the decision about what they will use.

COMMUNICATING WITH YOUR DOCTOR

While you could simply give your doctor the symptom sheet you completed, reducing this information to only the most important points is more effective as it will be shorter, more clear and easier to read.

Any written report should be no longer than 1 to 2 typed pages. Avoid providing a handwritten report, if possible. Doctors are busy and want only the most important information presented in the most concise, easy-to-read format. Bulleted lists often work well as they force you to be organized and brief, and provide high impact to the reader.

Suggested report format:

Your name, birth date (to ensure the correct file is accessed)

Dear Doctor ____________,

First paragraph - main concerns (the symptoms you really need fixed). "My main concerns are..." (for example heavy periods, hot flashes, low libido...)
Second paragraph - "I would like to discuss the possibility of trying following therapy at my appointment with you on day/month/year:" write what you believe you will benefit from, including the dosage if you know what it should be.

Third paragraph - "These are my symptoms, and what I understand they mean:" Follow with a bulleted list of symptoms, for example:

- Heavy periods with clots requiring tampon plus overnight pad
    - Suggests low progesterone
- Shortened cycle
    - Suggests low progesterone
- Breast soreness, fluid retention, large amount of clear vaginal mucous
    - Suggests high estrogen

Your doctor should be your partner in re-balancing your hormones and keeping you healthy and comfortable. With background knowledge, forethought and planning, and good communication about what therapy you want to try, you should be able to discuss all options with your doctor.

If you can, provide this information in writing a few days before your appointment to allow him or her to digest your information and request, and to seek further information or confirmation if necessary. Aim to keep the information you provide to your doctor on a single page, if at all possible, or two pages maximum. Like all busy professionals, they prefer communication that is clear, direct and "to the point".

CHAPTER EIGHT

IS SALIVA TESTING USEFUL?

Although blood testing is more readily available to physicians, saliva testing is another option accessible to patients themselves to confirm hormone levels, as a doctor's order is not needed and no expertise is required to collect a sample of saliva for testing. The downside is that often government and private insurances do not cover the cost, although it is certainly worthwhile checking your coverage to determine whether they will pay for these tests.

The problem with any single test, however, is that it is a "snapshot" in time, while our hormones are constantly cycling. Tracking hormone changes over time, with multiple tests, can be costly as well as inconvenient for the client. In my experience, women's symptoms and body signs that tell us what her hormones are doing usually give me more information than I can get from a single blood or saliva test.

However, in cases where the symptoms are not completely clear, testing can be useful. Testosterone, for example, is sometimes confusing. If a woman has low libido and fatigue but lacks other supporting symptoms such as decreased hair growth, we would hesitate to try supplemental testosterone without a test to verify that low testosterone is the source of the problem.

Keep in mind, some hormones need to be measured during a particular phase of the menstrual cycle when they are at their peak production. Measuring progesterone during menstruation, for example, would give little useful information as it is normally low at that point of the cycle. The preferred timing would be to test for progesterone a few days after ovulation is expected, when levels should be highest.

CHAPTER NINE

CASE STUDIES

Please note that all patient names are fictitious and that the patients themselves are composites of many I have seen with similar symptoms.

These cases also contain information on dosages and monitoring for effectiveness, plus other miscellaneous information that was not already covered. Please forgive a certain amount of repetition of information previously given – in some cases, it was necessary to present a complete picture of the thought process used to arrive at the chosen therapy.

Quotes attributed to clients are typical of what women would often say to me, but are not direct quotes from any particular person.

The Teenage Years

Hormone imbalances can occur at any age, not just during the menopausal change. The mom of a teenage girl we'll call Julie asks if they can come for an appointment together. Julie's mom tells me her daughter has been having very heavy flooding periods with painful cramping for over a year. Their doctor has tried her on several different types of birth control pills and, while they helped reduce flow and cramping, they also caused a number of side effects. She is wondering what else her daughter could try to control the problem.

Menstrual cycles begin, on average, around age 13 with age 8 to 18 being considered normal. Several factors are believed to influence the age of menarche (the first menstrual period), including genetics, percentage of body fat, exercise, nutrition, and possibly psychological and emotional factors. It has been noted that the age of menarche has decreased over the past century, and it has been suggested that environmental factors, with increased exposure to estrogen-like compounds, such as those contained in pesticides and plastics, may be contributing to earlier sexual development.

Similar to menopause when cycles are winding down, ovulation often does not occur regularly for many girls as cycles begin, leading to decreased progesterone production since a corpus luteum is not formed in cycles without ovulation. It is possible that the uncharacteristic moodiness accompanied by heavier periods that can occur during the teen years may be related to a resulting hormone imbalance, with a lack of progesterone being produced when ovulation does not occur. Progesterone actions tend to balance for or "oppose" the actions of estrogen, leading to the use of the term "unopposed estrogen" for a hormone imbalance when estrogen is produced without the normal cyclic production of progesterone. The dominance of estrogen, due to progesterone being missing, can lead to increased thickening of the endometrium (the lining of the uterus), breast soreness and fluid retention or "bloating" – common symptoms described as pre-menstrual syndrome or PMS. Progesterone also connects to the same benzodiazepine receptors that Valium activates, creating a calming effect on the brain, so decreased production relative to estrogen can be associated with anxiety and irritability in women of any age.

So, to go back to our client Julie, an alternative suggestion to birth control pills could be progesterone cream. Ideally, I would want to check signs and symptoms during an unmedicated cycle that would tell us if she was producing estrogen but not progesterone: heavy periods, premenstrual syndrome (fluid retention, bloating, moodiness in the week or 10 days before menstruation), and what color the menstrual fluid is at the beginning of her period. Pink or red is normal; brown flow at the beginning of the period signals the presence of unshed lining from the previous cycle, with a lack of progesterone that promotes complete shedding of the endometrial lining of the uterus. Birth control pills contain a synthetic progestin that would most likely improve the problem of heavy periods, but they also contain estrogen, adding to what she is already producing rather than correcting only the problem that exists. The additional estrogen or the use of a synthetic progestin rather than progesterone, the progestogen that her body normally produces, could be causing her unpleasant side effects.

I recommended starting her on 30mg of transdermal progesterone daily, starting on day 10 of her cycle and continuing until her period starts. The goal was to replace the normal amount of progesterone that should be produced, at the same time as it would normally be produced. The dose of progesterone would need to be enough to balance the (unknown) amount of estrogen that she was producing. Since every woman is different, the amount of estrogen being produced, and therefore the amount of progesterone needed, would vary. 30mg daily is an approximate production during the "luteal phase", between ovulation and the start of menstruation when the corpus luteum is active, so provides a starting point for dosing. I often recommend that women monitor the amount and quality of vaginal mucous being produced: Clear, lubricative (or "slippery") mucous indicates that estrogen is present without enough progesterone being produced to balance the estrogen; yellow or white creamy mucous indicates that sufficient progesterone is present to balance the estrogen. Larger amounts of clear, slippery mucous suggests higher levels of estrogen without progesterone. When dosing progesterone in the luteal phase, I would suggest increasing the dose of progesterone if clear slippery mucous is present, until the mucous dries up or changes to white or yellowish and creamy in texture.

Another alternative for our client, Julie, would be the herbal medicine, Vitex (also known as Chaste Berry). This herb encourages production of progesterone in the body and, when effective, would achieve the same result. I would recommend the same monitoring of symptoms as above to determine the effectiveness of the therapy when using Vitex.

Perimenopause

Marianne is a 47-year-old office worker who has attended one of my "lunch and learn" seminars on hormones. "I need help!" she said, when she called afterward to make an appointment with me. Like many women I see in their years leading up to menopause, she described extremely heavy periods and terrible PMS-like symptoms in the week before her period that had been getting worse over the last 2 years. The length of her periods and the interval between periods were varying wildly, unlike in earlier years when they were predictable and regular. Her menstrual flow was dark brown at the beginning, suggesting that the endometrial lining of the uterus had not completely shed the month before, and the flow contained a lot of blood clots. Both of these symptoms suggest low amounts of progesterone but plenty of estrogen were being produced. Progesterone blocks estrogen's effect of stimulating growth of the endometrium, resulting in less build-up of lining, and causes blood vessels in the endometrium to shrink leading to less actual blood loss and less likelihood of clotting. Normal menstrual fluid, although red in color, actually contains sloughed off glands and fluids but not a large amount of blood, so usually does not form clots.

Although many women do not realize it, the definition of "menopause" is actually the date of the last menstrual period. Everything else, including all the changes leading up to that last period, is called "perimenopause". Menopause has not officially occurred until a woman has been one full year without a menstrual period, and the date is then assigned retrospectively. So, a woman is technically in the perimenopause phase until the date of menopause is established. Once that year has passed with no bleeding, she is considered to have been "post-menopausal" from the date of her final menstrual period.

During the reproductive years, once regular cycles are established, hormones tend to cycle fairly regularly. Illness, high levels of stress or an emotional crisis can disrupt the cycle (most often causing a delay in ovulation and subsequently menstruation) but generally regular cycles will be re-established once the issue is resolved. The time between ovulations is consistent in most women with ovulation occurring 12 to 16 days before the next period starts. A delayed menstruation usually means ovulation was delayed and this can be caused by stress, illness or dieting - any situation where the body might sense that it was not a good time to become pregnant.

It is normal for the number of mucous production days before ovulation to gradually decrease as a woman ages, and this is one reason that fertility decreases with age. The wet mucous that occurs with rising estrogen levels before ovulation is necessary to enable sperm to move through the cervix, enabling exposure to a viable ovum (or egg).

As menopause approaches, during the perimenopause, the cycles may begin to change. The old textbook description of menopause describes how the event occurs when the ovaries run out of eggs, causing the cycles to stop. While this scenario still occurs, many women now notice several changes in the years before menopause, including a change in the length, quality and appearance of menstrual flow. Some women also experience a change in the number of days between menstrual periods, with the cycle becoming shorter. Often periods will be simply skipped as the menopause date approaches.

Canadian researcher, Dr. Jerilynn C. Prior, identified as many as 40% of perimenopausal women she studied who did not ovulate or ovulated and did not produce a normal amount of progesterone. This lack of production can lead to an unbalancing of estrogen and progesterone, resulting in "PMS-like" symptoms, such as fluid retention, mood changes, and breast soreness. As, described earlier, in a normal cycle, the ovary releases two hormones at ovulation, progesterone and inhibin, that trigger a down-regulation (or reduced activity) of the menstrual control center in the brain. (Inhibin is a less-studied hormone that inhibits production of hormones in the brain that stimulate the menstrual cycle).

If ovulation does not occur, progesterone and inhibin are not produced. This causes continued and increasing production of ovary-stimulating hormones by the brain (FSH and LH) as the control center in the brain tries to push the ovaries to produce an egg. These two hormones stimulate the ovaries, as they are supposed to, sometimes resulting in very high estrogen levels and little or no progesterone production when the ovary is still partially functioning in perimenopause.

Dr. Prior's research found that women could have estrogen levels as much as 6 to 7 times higher than normal, and called this "hyper-stimulated ovary syndrome". She noted that this hormone imbalance was not described in any of the medical texts she had studied in medical school, suggesting it is a newer phenomenon in women.

Some doctors simply test for increased blood levels of FSH and LH to diagnose that a woman has begun the menopausal change. However, these tests give no information about the levels of estrogen, progesterone and testosterone, the hormones that result in perimenopausal symptoms when not produced in proper, balanced amounts. To know how hormone production has changed, one would need to test for each of these hormones or analyze symptoms in detail.

Although blood or saliva tests for these hormones are useful, symptoms can often give us as good or sometimes better clues about what changes are happening to various hormone in the body. Any single blood test can only give a "snapshot" in time, and we know that hormone levels are constantly changing. However, if tests are done, it is important to test during the luteal phase (the time between ovulation and when the period starts) when progesterone is produced, and ideally in mid-luteal phase to catch peak production. This timing is necessary to detect whether ovulation occurred and if progesterone is being produced.

For many years, almost all women were given the same dosage and type of hormone replacement, regardless of their symptoms, so testing for individual hormones was thought to be unnecessary. With the passage of time, however, research has shown that these early hormone regimens caused more harm than good and they are infrequently prescribed now. You can imagine how administering more estrogen to a woman who already has several times higher than normal estrogen might lead to some unpleasant side effects, such as worsened fluid retention, weight gain and sore breasts. One simple rule of thumb used in Bioidentical Hormone Replacement Therapy is that if a woman is still having menstrual periods, she must be producing enough estrogen to create a thickened endometrium and therefore generally does not need additional estrogen.

For my client, Marianne, my questioning about her hormone related symptoms suggested that she was experiencing the "hyper-stimulated ovary syndrome" that was described by Dr. J. C. Prior, where a lack of progesterone production at ovulation was leading to increased production of FSH and LH, which in turn was stimulating her partially functioning ovaries to produce higher than normal levels of estrogen. This syndrome can begin at any age, and I have seen it in women as young as their 30's. Often these women were told they were too young to be perimenopausal.

By the time I saw Marianne, her estrogen was so high we needed to give a larger than normal dose of progesterone to balance the amount of estrogen she was producing. We also started it immediately after her period (rather than waiting until the expected time of ovulation at mid-cycle when natural production would begin) to prevent excessive buildup of the endometrial lining of the uterus that results in a heavier period as it sloughs off at the end of the cycle. We started with 40mg of progesterone daily, and I instructed her to increase the dose by 5mg daily if she observed any wet lubricative "estrogen" mucous the previous day, up to a maximum of 60mg daily (I've never had a client require more than 60mg daily).

Although the herbal medicine, Vitex, stimulates natural production of progesterone, it is questionable whether it could achieve enough production to balance very high level of estrogens. However, she could consider taking the herbal supplement DIM (Diindolylmethane) which encourages metabolism and clearing of estrogen from the body. DIM is also found in cruciferous vegetables, such as cabbage, broccoli, bok choy, Brussels sprouts, cauliflower, kale and turnip.

Surgical Menopause

Jane is a 44-year-old woman who had a hysterectomy, without removal of her ovaries, 3 years earlier due to large uterine fibroids. She was fine for 2 years, but then her ovaries started to fail (as sometimes occurs, within 1 to 2 years after surgery). An interruption in blood supply to the ovaries, a result of the surgery, is believed to cause this problem in some women. She began taking estrogen only, Premarin 0.625mg, and improved greatly. A progestogen was considered unnecessary, as she no longer had a uterus to protect. Now, however, after 1 year on Premarin, she finds she has new complaints. "I am so tired all the time! I'm not interested in things that I normally enjoy doing, and just forget about sex... I couldn't care less!", she told me.

After reviewing her hormone related symptoms, I could see a pattern emerging that suggested low testosterone. In addition to the fatigue, lack of sex drive and disinterest in activities she normally enjoyed, she also described notably reduced hair growth on legs, underarms and pubic area; decreased muscle strength; and a recent bone density test showed she had lost bone since her baseline test at the time of her surgery.

When hormones are given by mouth, they are immediately processed by the liver, as are all substances that are absorbed by our digestive systems. This is referred to in medicine as the "first pass effect". Essentially all drugs taken by mouth are passed through the liver when first absorbed, changing or eliminating part of the dose before the drug has a chance to act on the body.

Hormones are fat soluble, so do not mix easily with watery blood. Our bodies have devised methods of transporting fat soluble substances. For hormones, one way is to bind them to Sex Hormone Binding Globulin (SHBG), a protein produced by the liver. However, protein-bound hormones cannot leave the blood to act on body tissues as easily as those that are transported in other ways, for example, attached to red blood cells.

Oral hormones, or those taken by mouth, stimulate the liver to make more SHBG, our body's effort to reduce the effect of an accidental ingestion of hormones in our food. This increased SHBG protein, however, binds testosterone 10 times more strongly than estrogen, resulting in less free testosterone. The net result is that oral estrogen can cause symptoms of low testosterone, even if the same amount of testosterone is being produced as before supplementation was started. However, much of our testosterone is produced by the ovaries so, in Jane's case, she could be producing less testosterone because her ovaries are failing, as well as having a larger percentage bound to the increased SHBG proteins that she is producing because of her oral estrogen supplement.

In the short term, to relieve her symptoms sooner, I suggested starting testosterone replacement. Testosterone is known to cause liver problems when given by mouth but, like other hormones, it is readily absorbed through the skin, so it makes sense to administer it in cream form, or "transdermally". While there are several transdermal testosterone products available on the market now, they are all dosed for men and are very expensive, as compared to the cost of the ingredients - often over $100 for ingredients that cost less than $10. Unfortunately, many women are prescribed these products and risk overdose, resulting in side effects such as facial hair growth and acne, because they have no way to measure an accurate dose.

I received a call from a woman in a nearby city who was using testosterone cream. She had broken out in severe acne and was wondering if her supplement could be causing the problem. A quick calculation, using the strength and amount of cream she was using, revealed she was applying 100mg of testosterone daily – a large dose even for a man! Had she continued this dose, she would likely have developed facial hair and eventually a change in her voice. When dosed properly for a woman, at 1mg or less a day with perhaps 2mg daily initially for a week or two to achieve results more quickly, women never experience these side effects. I instructed her to stop the supplement completely until the acne cleared, and to speak to her pharmacist about reducing the dose to 1mg daily when she restarted.

For my client, Jane, I also suggested progesterone replacement, given as a transdermal cream and used cyclically, for 2 weeks of each month. Because of the historical reason for the introduction of a progestogen to hormone replacement therapy, to protect the uterine endometrium from overgrowth, progesterone is virtually never offered to women who have had a hysterectomy. And, of course, since the synthetic progestin, medroxyprogesterone, is really designed only to protect the uterus, it doesn't make sense to prescribe it to these women, since they have no uterus to protect!

But real progesterone acts in areas other than the uterus, and the rest of a woman's body would benefit from supplementation if it is lacking. It is not reasonable to think a hormone would act on only one tissue of the body. And, in Jane's case, progesterone would also provide her with a source of hormones to replace what her failing ovaries could no longer produce since it can be changed by her body into other hormones including testosterone as needed.

Progesterone also stimulates the body to create more estrogen receptors, increasing the effectiveness of a dose of estrogen. Dr. John Lee (Natural Progesterone – The Multiple Actions of a Remarkable Hormone) observed that his patients who were already taking estrogen alone could usually reduce their dose by half when progesterone was started.

As with testosterone, I would suggest administering the progesterone transdermally. Progesterone also passes easily through the skin and, as explained earlier, it is highly metabolized by the liver as soon as it is absorbed. The transdermal dose used is generally about 1/10th of the oral dose. Ninety percent of swallowed progesterone is changed into metabolites that connect to benzodiazepine receptors in the brain. Diazepam, brand name Valium, is a well-known drug in the benzodiazepine class; others include alprazolam, triazolam, and flurazepam. These benzodiazepine drugs are used as tranquilizers and sleeping pills, so it is easy to understand why excessive drowsiness is one of the main side effects of oral progesterone. When given transdermally, in amounts normally produced by the body during a regular cycle, progesterone does not cause drowsiness.

Another option for Jane, that might eliminate the need for additional testosterone, would be to change to transdermal estrogen, using either a compounded cream or a commercially available estrogen patch or gel. This change would achieve several advantages: her estrogen dose would be much lower (like other hormones, estrogen is metabolized on its first pass through the liver), she would eliminate the increased risk of gall bladder disease associated with oral estrogen, and she would avoid increased production of SHBG protein that is "tying up" a large percentage of her own testosterone. This would reduce her need for a testosterone supplement. Adding progesterone would not only balance the actions of administered estrogen throughout her body, it would also give her a source of testosterone, as progesterone can be converted into testosterone, estrogen and other hormones in the body. So, with progesterone as part of her hormone replacement, Jane may not need testosterone and could require a lower estrogen dose.

Medicine is not an exact science – some physicians describe it as often being as much art as science. There are often multiple ways to address a woman's hormone imbalance, as you see above, and I discuss these options with my clients to determine their preferences for therapy. Sometimes, we try one approach but keep the others as options, depending on her response to the first choice.

Postmenopause

Anna is a 52-year-old woman who provides training sessions for a large corporation. Her periods stopped 13 months ago. She is well read in health issues and is aware of the controversy about standard hormone therapy. She had been managing her menopausal symptoms with lifestyle, diet and exercise, but finds that in recent months symptoms have gotten out of control, especially the hot flashes. "It's worst when I get up in front of a group to give a presentation, and that's what I do for a living! I actually bring a change of clothes, so I'll have something dry to put on afterward...", she tells me.

As the ovaries are winding down, hormone production can become erratic. For many years, clinicians have explained the cause of hot flashes as a lack of estrogen; however, newer research where hormone levels were actually measured during a hot flash showed it is a drop in estrogen and not a true lack of hormone that brings on the flushing and sweats. Even women with higher than normal estrogen, described in the "hyper-stimulated ovary" syndrome in the perimenopause case study, would experience hot flashes when their levels dropped from 6 times higher than normal to 4 times higher!

As hormone production becomes more erratic, the menstrual control center in the brain also becomes more reactive, leading to varying levels of stimulation of ovaries with resulting swings in hormone production.

Assessment of Anna's symptoms suggested that her hormones are relatively in balance but fluctuating, as often happens during the menopausal change. The most troublesome time for her, though, was when she has the extra stress of speaking to an audience. Stress hormones, that are often produced when we are under pressure, have a structure somewhat similar to our reproductive hormones and can block hormone receptors, giving the effect of a decrease in hormones. Anna's symptoms did not include vaginal dryness, so I concluded that her estrogen was likely not excessively low, although she was no longer having menstrual periods. I therefore suggested a very low amount of estrogen in cream form from the 4th of each calendar month until the end of the month, along with progesterone 30mg in cream form from the 14th to the end of the month to provide a stable amount of hormone in her system. Although we could have used daily administration, there is some evidence that cyclic administration that mimics natural production may be best for bone health.

I instructed her to always measure the cream for consistency, and pre-loaded it into syringes (without a needle) to make this easier. She was happy to start with a low dose and use cyclic administration because she was interested in using the least amount of medication necessary. I recommended only hormones that were already being produced by her body: estriol, a weak estrogen for balance, and estradiol a stronger estrogen to ensure adequate effect, in an 80:20 ratio, with natural progesterone to balance or "oppose" the negative effects of estrogen. I instructed her to begin with 0.5mg of the BiEst 80:20 and to increase her dose by 0.1mg once a month until she was experiencing adequate relief of her symptoms. Progesterone would be dosed as 30mg daily on days 14 (of the calendar) to the end of the month. A hormone-free break for the first 3 days of the month was recommended to maintain the activity of the hormones. Similar to staring at a bright light and being unable to see in semi-darkness afterward for a short period of time (caused by fatigue of the vision receptors in the eye), hormone receptors can become "fatigued" by being exposed to a constant source of hormones.

In women whose symptoms were controlled with higher doses of hormone, for example 60mg of progesterone daily, and were complaining of a return of symptoms after several months, I recommend stopping treatment completely for 2 weeks with monitoring for improvement or deterioration of symptoms to confirm a suspected excessive dose. The woman would then be restarted at a lower dose.

In women who describe themselves as "desperate", "can't stand it any more" or "need this problem fixed NOW", I might take a different approach, starting at the higher end of the normal dose range and giving instructions to decrease the dose very gradually once symptoms are under control. I believe that discussion about how the client wants to approach treatment is an important part of any medical consultation. A paternalistic approach of "this is how I have decided to treat you" with no discussion is rapidly becoming less acceptable in many treatment situations. Educating patients in their options and involving them in treatment decision making, as much as possible, often results in better treatment adherence (or "sticking with the treatment plan") and better results from the treatment.

For Anna, I also suggested that she start a B-Complex-100 tablet once daily in the morning. B vitamins, in particular Pantothenic Acid, also known as vitamin B5, will sometimes reduce the amount of stress hormones produced. Since her hot flashes were worst when she was under stress, controlling and "evening out" her stress hormone production during the day would most likely help reduce her main complaint of hot flashes during presentations.

The composition of compounded estrogen cream...

The original formula of compounded estrogen cream was called TriEstrogen and contained the 3 main estrogens produced by women's bodies: estriol 80%, estrone 10% and estradiol 10%, based on what was then believed to be the natural ratio of these estrogens in the body. Estradiol is the strongest form of estrogen, estrone is a storage form of estrogen, and estriol is the weakest estrogen. Estriol is considered to be a safer and "balancing" estrogen, as it does not stimulate breast or endometrial tissues, and does not increase clotting of the blood, but still has a positive effect on vaginal tissue, hot flashes and possibly bone (although study results vary on this). The second estrogen, estrone, has been dropped from the formula by many compounders because of the development of a negative regard for estrone since the body can store and change it back to the stronger estradiol at a later time. Interestingly, virtually all swallowed estradiol is changed into estrone, and women taking oral estradiol generally have much higher than normal levels of estrone. This desire to reduce estrone resulted in the formula: estriol 80%, estradiol 20%, and often is referred to as BiEstrogen 80/20.

The 80/20 or 80/10/10 ratios of compounded estrogen are also being questioned in some circles, with a 50/50 ratio of estriol to estradiol being suggested as more similar to the natural balance produced in the female body, based on more recent testing. It is considered important in BHRT to have some weak estriol administered along with progesterone whenever estradiol is given, as naturally occurs in the body. This is important to balance the action of the stronger estradiol, which gives sufficient estrogen activity for relief of symptoms. Converting the commonly used doses of 0.5 to 1mg of TriEstrogen 80/10/10 (or BiEstrogen 80/20) to BiEstrogen 50/50 would equate roughly to 0.2 to 0.4mg of total estrogen daily, if the amount of estradiol is kept consistent. In a woman with more severe symptoms who was anxious for quick results or who was converting from standard hormone therapy, I might start with up to 2mg of total estrogen daily of BiEstrogen 80/20 (0.8mg of BiEst 50/50 to obtain an equal amount of estradiol, the stronger estrogen) and gradually reduce the dose.

The creams can be made in any strength; what is important is to know the concentration of hormone in the cream, and to carefully measure the amount that will give the dose of hormone needed, titrating gradually to the lowest amount that will relieve symptoms. Sometimes women wanted their cream "as strong as possible" but the important factor is the amount measured, not how many milligrams (mg) per milliliter (ml) of hormone it contains. A preparation of 1 mg of estrogen in each ml (usually written as "1 mg/ml") would simplify calculation of the dose. Pharmacists make progesterone cream, which is used in higher milligram doses than estrogen, in varying mg/ml strengths. I have usually made 100mg/ml (or 10%), again to make calculation of the dose easier. In USA, progesterone is commonly available as a 2% cream (20mg/ml) in health food stores and some pharmacies.

Many women use progesterone doses of 20 to 60mg daily, so the corresponding doses would be 0.2 to 0.6ml daily if using a product that contained 100mg/ml of progesterone. Depending on the graininess of the progesterone powder that your pharmacist is able to obtain, they may only be able to prepare a lower strength, such as 2% or 20mg/ml, to avoid grittiness in the final product, unless they have specialized compounding equipment, specifically an ointment mill, to smooth the final product. Any grittiness would indicate particles of progesterone that would be too large to pass through the skin, resulting in a lowered effective dose. The end result is the same, however, if the appropriate quantity is measured to give the desired milligram daily dose. With a 2% (20mg/ml) cream a 20 to 60mg dose would be 1 to 3ml.

I am a Canadian pharmacist. In Canada, all hormones require a prescription. As I understand US regulations, federal law allows some hormones in cream form to be sold without prescription in different strengths, but state regulations may prevent pharmacists from selling it without a prescription (depending on the laws of the individual state). This has resulted in a strange situation where you may be able to buy progesterone cream in a health food store, but not a pharmacy. Unfortunately, some non-prescription products do not indicate the amount of progesterone in each milliliter. I would recommend that you only buy a product that has the strength indicated on the label and measure it carefully every day to ensure you are using a consistent amount.

When talking to your doctor about your use of a non-prescription product, it is ideal to tell him how many milligrams of progesterone you use daily to give you best results, so he will understand exactly what you are using. A syringe without a needle is simple to fill with most creams and will give you an accurate measurement if you can avoid air bubbles. You can ask your pharmacist for an empty syringe of 1 to 3 ml. Alternatively, you could use a 1- or 2-ml measuring spoon, being sure to level the measurement. However, spoons tend to be less accurate and it is more difficult to make small adjustments to the dosage than with a syringe.

Vaginal Dryness

Janice is an older woman, well past the menopause change at age 65. "Can I speak to you in private?", she asks me. "Of course," I answer, and take her into my private consultation room. "This is so embarrassing." she begins. But I assure her that pharmacists are trained to keep everything said to them completely confidential.

She describes terrible vaginal dryness that has been bothersome for over a year. She has tried several non-prescription lubricants, but nothing seems to help. "It's gotten so bad now that having sex with my husband has become very uncomfortable" she tells me. "I'm worried that it's starting to have an effect on our marriage - you know, he thinks I'm just not interested and I guess I'm really not, since it's not enjoyable for me any more."

We decide to book an appointment, so I will have time to review her symptoms thoroughly. Vaginal atrophy (or thinning of the vaginal tissues) causing discomfort during sex is her main complaint, and this is generally believed to be due to low levels of estrogen. For some women, using a sterile lubricant before sexual activity, such as KY Jelly (or a generic equivalent), solves the problem. There is also a higher-level lubricant called Replens that is designed to bind to the inside of the vagina, staying there for several days. It that can also be more helpful when symptoms of dryness or irritation are noticed at other times as well.

Increasing the amount of foreplay can also give a woman's body more time to produce her own lubricating fluids. Being well hydrated is important too - it's more difficult to produce fluids if you're dehydrated.

This client has tried these strategies did not find them sufficiently helpful. However, she also describes other signs of low hormone production, including low muscle mass, fatigue and body hair loss that suggest low testosterone levels. Low testosterone in women is widely believed to contribute to a lack of interest in sex, but some clinicians do not realize that it can also be a cause of vaginal dryness.

So, for Janice, the situation is not as clear as it often can be. She has expressed a desire to use the minimum dose of hormones, and only if necessary. "I didn't need them to get through menopause", she tells me, "and I don't want to start now unless I really need to."

Blood tests for estradiol (the strongest estrogen and the one that is usually measured), and for "free" testosterone (to avoid including testosterone that is bound to proteins in the blood and is therefore inactive), would give a valuable clue as to which hormone (or possibly both) is lacking and causing Janice's problem. Saliva tests could also be done - hormones are excreted into saliva and are easily measured, but this test is only done at one Canadian lab as far as I am aware, and is not covered by provincial Medicare as yet, making it less attractive for some clients, although a few private insurances may cover the tests. In US, a woman would need to check with her health insurance provider to determine coverage. There are several American companies that do saliva hormone tests. Most companies, both in Canada and US, provide a sample collection kit that can be ordered by phone or through their website, and is received and returned by regular mail. It is a useful type of testing to be aware of as a doctor's order is not necessary and the women herself can request the test.

After discussing the options, together we decide that asking her doctor for blood tests and making a decision based on the results is the route she would like to take. Other options we considered were to try a standard low-dose estradiol suppository or a compounded estriol gel (the weak natural estrogen that is highly effective at restoring the vaginal lining); a trial of low dose testosterone replacement in cream form (2mg per day until effect, then reducing to 1mg per day); or progesterone cream 30mg a day.

Progesterone is considered a very safe hormone - during pregnancy women produce 300 to 400mg a day, and pregnancy is associated with less risk of cancer not increased risk. It is also a "precursor" hormone that can be changed into other hormones as needed in the body, so it could become a supply of either estrogen or testosterone, or both. Estriol is also the main estrogen produced during pregnancy and is considered a safe estrogen for this reason as well as the fact that it is not metabolized into other, stronger estrogens but stays in its weak form until eliminated from the body. Of course, using only estriol would not address any testosterone deficiency she might have.

In response to my report, Janice's doctor ordered the hormone blood tests, which showed she was low in both estradiol and testosterone. To improve her problem more quickly, and in accordance with Janice's desire to use the safest approach possible, we decided to ask her doctor to prescribe estriol vaginal gel (1mg of estriol inserted at bedtime until improvement, then decreased to 0.5mg at bedtime until reassessment). I suggested a gel rather than a cream, as the gel form is more similar to natural vaginal fluids and would provide superior lubricative qualities. We also asked for a prescription for progesterone 30mg daily, as transdermal cream, to provide a source of both estrogen and testosterone for long-term supplementation. After one month, she reduced the dose of vaginal estriol to 0.5mg and was able to discontinue it after 3 months, as the progesterone was being metabolized into sufficient estrogen and testosterone for her needs.

Transgender

I have had the great privilege to work with a few transgender clients over the years. It has helped me to realize gender is a more fluid state than I once thought - more of a spectrum and not "black and white" as many believe. The idea of feeling uncomfortable with the gender assigned to you at birth may be foreign to many of us, but perhaps this is the best way to understand it: Gender, it seems, is not determined by the physical traits of the body, but in the brain. When the two don't match, it can create great emotional conflict for an individual. Fortunately, today's society is much more open to new understanding.

Having a clinic pharmacy that was more like an office than a store, especially back in the 90's, was truly amazing. I was able to have very private conversations that clients would never have initiated in a regular pharmacy. One client told me he had been raised as a boy, but at puberty he had started to develop as a woman. He said his doctors discovered that he had a combination of male and female reproductive organs. His parents and his doctors had had a discussion and determined the best route of action was for him to undergo surgery to prevent the female development that was starting to take place. Apparently, no one thought to ask his opinion of what should be done. "I've always felt more like a girl than a boy", he told me, "but I wasn't asked what I thought the doctors should do".

Now, in his mid-20s, he was seeing specialists in another city to correct what he felt was a mistake made when he was in his early teens. I think it helped him to talk about his situation, and I felt privileged that he was comfortable talking about it with me. He would be required to live as a woman for at least 1 year before any surgery would be considered, and he would have regular visits with a psychologist to help him cope with the inevitable stress he would endure with such a dramatic life change.

I came into contact with another transgender client much later in her journey. She contacted me because she wanted to use a more natural estrogen combination than was available commercially. Beginning as apparently male, but with a strong feeling that she needed to become a woman, she had already undergone surgery and it was a tall, beautiful woman that I met with to discuss how we could fine-tune her hormones.

She was working with a local endocrinologist, and I think we were both surprised at how well she could sense when she needed more or less estrogen. Not surprisingly, she required more than most women, and we allowed her to determine her ideal amount of estrogen herself, according to her response. I also made her estrogen cream in a higher strength to reduce the volume she needed to apply daily.

It can be difficult to understand the journey others have chosen or are compelled to take, but I felt my role was to understand as best I could, and to help to the best of my ability. I found that I learned a great deal on many levels from my clients.

CHAPTER TEN

THOUGHTS FOR THE FUTURE

In compounding circles, the importance of the "Triad" of care is often discussed. This Triad refers to you, your pharmacist and your doctor. All three should be working together to solve problems you may encounter and to keep you healthy.

I was told once that the name "physician" was derived from the word for "teacher". Physicians were people who taught us how to be healthy. These days, however, many doctors seem too busy simply trying to fix health problems, so who has taken over the task of teaching us what to do to be healthy?

Pharmacists have been expanding their roles in the healthcare system in recent years. You may have noticed that some pharmacists can now prescribe for minor ailments or order tests and continue your prescription when you are unable to see your doctor. Most can now administer some immunizations as well, such as flu shots or vaccines that are recommended before taking a trip and, in some jurisdictions, give birth control, heparin and other injections that are given in the arm. Many are also doing medication reviews and other services by appointment. Others are doing diabetes counseling or hormone consultations, similar to what I have done for many years.

It seems that many health problems could be corrected or even prevented if people had knowledge of changes that would create a healthier lifestyle. It is so unfortunate that many of our physicians no longer have the time for this teaching role, with many allowing clients to only discuss one or two "problems" at each visit due to time constraints.

I believe that pharmacists are in an ideal position to assume the role of teaching clients how to stay healthy and how to reduce their risk factors for various diseases. In many areas of the country, there is a shortage of doctors and this, along with assessing and prescribing for minor ailments, would be a logical way to create increased physician time to treat more complex cases where a higher level of expertise is needed. Nurses are another logical group who could expand their services into disease prevention, but pharmacists have the advantage of already having facilities in the community and daily contact with clients who are seeking advice on non-prescription drugs and prescriptions. I believe this is one reason why I started receiving the requests for information that lead me to specialize in hormone management - I was there and it was easy for women to contact me. Some women just dropped in to my pharmacy and asked questions to find out how I could help them - interviewing me for the job, so to speak...

If you are looking for further information on any health condition, ask your pharmacist whether they offer in-depth counselling on hormone imbalances, or have considered doing so, and if not, whether they can refer you to a colleague who does!

My goal, with this book, has been to increase women's understanding of hormone imbalances and their options for correcting them, and thereby to help improve their quality of life. Providing women with good information can enable them to have a full discussion of treatment options with their doctors. Women have the right to understand what is happening to their bodies, and this understanding can help women, themselves, take control of their health, especially at a time when things can seem out of control. Knowledge can give us strength, power and a sense of control.

APPENDIX I

PROGESTERONE INFORMATION

BIOIDENTICAL (NATURAL) PROGESTERONE INFORMATION
JEANNIE COLLINS BEAUDIN, Pharmacist
jeannie.beaudin@gmail.com

When progesterone cream was removed from the shelves in Canada in the mid-90's due to being reclassified as prescription status, several women who were using it asked if I could supply them. When I found no products were available in Canada and I could not order it from US as these American products had not been approved for sale by Health Canada, I offered to compound it for them (pharmacists have an exemption to prepare products under a physician's order without having Health Canada approval). It is noteworthy that progesterone cream is considered safe enough by American regulators to be sold without a prescription in US. Since I was making the cream and because the clients using it had questions I could not answer, I began reading books and researching journal articles on the subject. I subsequently attended two seminars on Bio-identical hormones in US and several in Canada.

In the course of my research, I have compiled a number of scientific articles that support the use of progesterone in cream form. I found data to support the absorption of progesterone through the skin (provided certain criteria are met),16 its action on breast tissue,17 its action on bone metabolism18 (although other studies

---

[16] . Weichers, J.W., "Barrier Function of the Skin in Relation to Percutaneous Absorption of Drugs". Pharmaceutisch Weekblad Scientific Edition, 11-1989.

[17] . Chang, K., et al, "Influences of Percutaneous Administration of Estradiol and Progesterone on Human Breast Eipthelial Cell Cycle in Vivo", Fertility and Sterility, April 1996, Vol.68, No.4, p.785-791.

question this action on bone),19 and its choice over synthetic progestins.20 As well, I have accumulated a library of books on the subject. A bibliography of available texts and copies of these articles are available on request.

PROGESTERONE DOSING INFORMATION

Normal cyclic production of progesterone in women is in the range of 20 to 30mg/day. In pregnancy, production increases to 300 to 400mg/day, so it has a wide safety margin. The goal of supplemental therapy would be to deliver a dose within this range. We have patients using 20 to 100mg per day transdermally, with 30 to 60mg being most common. By comparison, oral progesterone which is highly metabolized by the liver, is dosed as 100 to 300mg daily. The high levels of progesterone metabolites produced cause the drowsiness that is noted with oral progesterone. Since progesterone is known to increase receptor sensitivity to estrogens, most women on estrogen-only therapy will need to reduce their estrogen dose when progesterone is added. Also, because of this increased estrogen receptor sensitivity, some women have adequate relief from hot flashes and other symptoms generally attributed to insufficient or fluctuating estrogen levels by using progesterone alone. In post-menopausal patients, it is recommended to have a hormone-free period of 4 to 7 days per month to maintain hormone activity. Pre-menopausal patients would normally supplement only during the luteal phase of the cycle. Progesterone would only be used throughout the cycle in pre-menopausal patients who were producing unusually high amounts of estrogen, a situation that is becoming more common.21

Although some authorities seem to assume 100% transdermal absorption while others estimate as low as 10%, the actual percentage is probably somewhere in between and variable according to the person's individual characteristics as well as the characteristics of the product base. Absorption has been shown to be consistent within an individual, although it can vary from person to person and correlates with

---

[18] . Prior, J.C., "Progesterone as a bone-trophic hormone". Endocrine Rev.,11(2):386-98, May 1990.

[19] . Leonetti HB, et al, "Transdermal progesterone cream for vasomotor symptoms and postmenopausal bone loss", Obstet Gynecol, Aug 1999; 94(2):225-8.

[20] . Schairer, C. , "Menopausal Estrogen and Estrogen-Progestin Replacement Therapy and Breast Cancer Risk". JAMA, Jan 26,2000, Vol.283,No.4.

[21] . Prior, J.C., "Perimenopause – The ovary's frustrating grand finale", A Friend Indeed, Vol xiv, No 7, Dec97/Jan98.

the transdermal absorption of other hormones, such as estradiol.22 We assume absorption of 80 to 90% with a properly milled product that is prepared in a proper base.

FACTORS THAT CAN INFLUENCE THE AMOUNT OF PROGESTERONE PASSING THROUGH THE SKIN:

- Site of application (areas of thinner skin may facilitate penetration)
- The vehicle in which the progesterone is applied (mineral oil can decrease absorption as it binds strongly to progesterone)
- Total surface area to which the cream is applied (larger area may result in more consistent blood levels)
- Skin condition (various factors such as presence of skin disease, mechanical or chemical damage to skin, occlusion, temperature)
- Skin age (although not well-proven, it is generally assumed that the skin of the young and the elderly is more permeable than adult tissue)

Progesterone and estrogen are well suited to absorption through the skin due to their low molecular weight and lipid solubility, and there are commercial preparations of transdermal patches and gels now being sold. In the application of progesterone in cream form, the skin acts as a reservoir, maintaining blood levels at a more constant level than many other forms of drug delivery, such as sublingual, oral and rectal. Progesterone, being lipid soluble, does not travel freely dissolved in aqueous blood but must be bound to red blood cells, proteins or lipid molecules, called chylomicrons.

The actual dose for each person will vary, due to individual variations in requirement, absorption and metabolism. There are many inter-related factors that come into play:

- Increased estrogens, in particular orally administered estrogens, which go directly to the liver on absorption, increase protein production by the liver, including sex hormone binding globulin (SHBG), which binds to estrogen, progesterone and testosterone causing decreased amounts of hormone free to act on tissues.
- Skin contains an enzyme, 5-alpha-reductase that occurs in varying amounts in different individuals, which can metabolize progesterone to

[22] . Burry KA, et al, "Percutaneous absorption of progesterone in postmenopausal women treated with transdermal estrogen", Am J Pbstet Gynedol, June 1999; 180(6 Pt 1):1504-11.

different degrees as it is absorbed, depending on the amount present. "Hairy" individuals tend to have higher levels of this enzyme in their skin.

- Progesterone, being lipid-soluble, is stored in fatty tissues in the body. When progesterone replacement is started in individuals who have been deficient for a period of time the fatty tissues will initially take up progesterone at a greater rate, leading to decreased progesterone activity when treatment is first started. Some sources suggest doubling the dose for the first 2 months to compensate for this.
- Discontinuing administration of progesterone for a short period of time each month is recommended by some authorities even after menopause to maintain receptor sensitivity.
- Estrogen is also thought to "prime" progesterone receptors; if lacking in progesterone effect when using this hormone alone, adding a small amount of estrogen may be necessary, although the body can convert progesterone to estrogen. Menstrual cycles can only occur with a blood estrogen level above 50pg/ml which is also considered to be the lower level goal in estrogen replacement therapy (50-150pg/ml). If menstrual cycles are occurring the woman would need to have adequate estrogen levels already and estrogen supplementation would be unnecessary.

Some clinicians prefer to measure saliva levels of progesterone as these levels represent more accurately the levels of free progesterone, as compared to blood levels that include progesterone bound to protein that is not biologically active. However, saliva tests are not processed at our local hospital and are therefore not covered by Medicare here in New Brunswick. The website of the Canadian saliva test lab is www.ramlab.com and that of the parent company, ZRT Laboratory, which has an extensive reference section is www.salivatest.com .

HOW TO MONITOR FOR EFFECT

- Relief of symptoms such as premenstrual water retention and weight gain, hot flashes, vaginal dryness.
- Bone scan (an increase in bone density would confirm adequate dose, but this would require at least a year of treatment)
- Drowsiness is a symptom of excessive transdermal dosage which is easy to monitor (drowsiness is expected with oral progesterone and may be helpful for insomnia.
- The type and amount of vaginal mucous produced (wet mucous indicates unopposed estrogen).

APPENDIX II

GENERAL BHRT INFORMATION

BIOIDENTICAL HORMONE REPLACEMENT
INFORMATION
Jeannie Collins Beaudin, Pharmacist

When I first heard about bioidentical hormone replacement, particularly administered through the skin in the form of a cream, I thought that it couldn't be valid since there were no commercial versions available in Canada. When I continued to receive questions from clients, along with requests to compound products (mostly transdermal) that were not available, I started researching, reading books and journal articles. I eventually attended two conferences in US and several in Canada and joined a network of compounding pharmacists, so I would have good answers for these women. One of the things I learned is that bioidentical hormones, being natural substances, cannot be patented in US. Therefore, there is little incentive to American pharmaceutical companies to do research and product development. In Canada, a prescription is required for all reproductive hormones, and a lot more documentation is necessary to bring a prescription product to market. That is very likely the main reason for the lack of information and commercial products available to us in Canada. Progesterone cream, estriol cream and estradiol cream are available without prescription in US, mainly in health food stores. Pharmacists, however, recognizing the monitoring that should occur in women using supplemental hormones, generally require a prescription. This surprising difference may be due to differing federal and state regulations.

CAN I SPEAK TO THE HORMONE LADY?

I am currently a retired pharmacist. My interest is to provide information on effective alternative treatments for women with menopausal complaints. As a compounding pharmacist, I prepared products from USP standardized ingredients for replacement of the three main classes of hormones used in women, the estrogens, progesterone and testosterone. For estrogen replacement, I made oral as well as transdermal forms, but the transdermal estrogens were the most popular, as stomach upset is avoided and lower doses of the potent forms of estrogen are needed. It is possible to make hormone replacement as sublingual drops as well, if that is a woman's preference.

Most women use one of two formulas we refer to as TriEstrogen (80% estriol, 10% estradiol and 10% estrone) or BiEstrogen (80% estriol and 20% estradiol) that attempt to maintain the natural balance of strong and weak circulating estrogens produced before menopause. I commonly made a preparation of 1mg total estrogen per ml and I always recommend that women measure the cream with a syringe for an accurate dose. I find that most women who have not previously taken hormones do well with 0.5 to 1mg daily but those who are switching from Premarin require much higher doses, 2 to 2.5mg daily. Interestingly, a study sponsored by Wyeth-Ayerst several years ago found good control of menopausal symptoms and fewer side effects with 0.3 to 0.45mg of Premarin than with the most commonly used 0.625mg strength. I expected that the recommended doses would be lowered but didn't notice any change after the study was released. It appears that the study was not well publicized. Another reason for lack of uptake of this new information may have been that many studies use Premarin 0.625mg, leaving the effectiveness of the 0.3mg on areas such as bone preservation, for example, untested.

Transdermal progesterone was the first bioidentical hormone replacement I began dispensing. Many postmenopausal women do well with only progesterone, as it increases the number of estrogen receptors and thereby improves the action of endogenous estrogens to sufficient levels. Progesterone can also be metabolized into estrogen, testosterone and other hormones, providing a supply of several hormones.

The other situation where I have found progesterone-only therapy to be valuable is with perimenopausal women who are having anovulatory cycles. Studies by Dr. Jerilynn Prior at UBC and others have found that significant percentages of women in their 40's do not ovulate regularly, with a resultant lack of progesterone being produced during the luteal phase of the cycle. In significant percentages of these women, the hypothalamus responds by causing the pituitary to release higher levels of FSH resulting in increased production of estrogen (measured as much as 6 to 7 times higher than normal) and in some women increased testosterone is also released by the ovary. This sets them up for the heavy flow, mood swings, increased PMS, etc., all signs of a domination of estrogen effect throughout the cycle, that conventional medicine tries to control with birth control pills containing a synthetic progestin plus more estrogen.

The dominating effect of the progestin in the pill usually fixes the problem with heavy bleeding but does nothing or may worsen other symptoms, such as breast soreness, fluid retention and mood problems. I found that replacing the progesterone from ovulation until menstruation in an amount sufficient to overcome signs of high estrogen works very well without further increasing their estrogen levels. I generally would suggest that they monitor for the disappearance of estrogen stimulated "eggwhite" vaginal mucous to gauge the amount needed.

I realize that many clinicians use this therapy approach with medroxyprogesterone, but I have seen three studies now in addition to the well-known Women's Health Initiative study, finding significantly increased rates of breast cancer with this drug and often have received complaints of breast tenderness from women using the therapy.

Oral progesterone represents an improvement in side-effect profile for many women, but the dose needs to be 8 to 10 times higher than when administered transdermally, due to metabolism during the first pass through the liver. Side effects such as drowsiness are attributed to the many metabolites produced, not to the progesterone itself. Women using the transdermal form of progesterone do not experience drowsiness and will often report clearer thinking and better memory function.

Transdermal testosterone has been used in women for years, as available oral commercial products are 10 to 20 times the strength needed, being designed for men. However, instead of a petrolatum base I recommend using a proper transdermal base and loading the cream into syringes to ensure it will be correctly measured. For women, a maintenance replacement dose is equal to 0.1ml or less of 1% strength – a very tiny amount that will deliver 1mg of testosterone. I do recommend that they start with 0.2 to 0.4ml daily until they notice some effect, however, to get things started, usually for a maximum of 2 weeks.

I have also noticed that excessive production of stress hormones, structurally similar to estrogen, is a significant contributor to menopausal symptoms and sleep disturbances. As our standard medical system has little to offer for controlling the effects of stress hormones, I have often suggested herbal medications or nutrients that have some evidence of benefit in this area. Phosphatidyl Serine is believed to lower cortisol production and can be useful for correcting some sleep disturbances; vitamin C and B Complex are involved in the production of cortisol; and several herbs, termed "adaptogens" can reduce the impact of excess cortisol on the body. It is interesting that the effects of cortisol are similar to the cluster of conditions we refer to as "Metabolic Syndrome".

APPENDIX III

HORMONE WORKSHEET

HORMONE CONSULT Payment discussed________

Name_______________________________
Date_________________________________
Phone_____________________________
Birthdate___________________________
Address___________________________
Doctor_____________________________
___________________________________Email or fax__________________

Current medications

____

____

Regular periods? __________________
Length________________________________
Frequency__________________________
Description____

____

Other cyclic symptoms

____

____

Pregnancies__________
Miscarriages____________________
Difficulty in getting pregnant? ____
Surgeries________________________

Main Concerns _______
____
____

SYMPTOMS
Hot flashes____
Night sweats____
Vaginal dryness/mucous___________________________________
Urinary symptoms____
Insomnia____
Fluid retention____
Breast soreness____
Weight gain____
Headaches ____
Heart palpitations____
Fatigue ____
Memory change____
Moods____
Hair loss/growth____
Bone loss____
Decreased muscle/cramps/aching___________________________
Low libido____
Joint pains/arthritis______________________________________
Bowel function____
Body temp/BP____
Stress____

GOALS AND ASSESSMENT
____
____
____

READING LIST

The following is a reading list that covers several important aspects of hormone function and imbalances in women:

Natural Progesterone: The Multiple Roles of a Remarkable Hormone

- Dr. John Lee, author
- Older text, but the definitive text on progesterone, written from Dr. Lee's clinical experiences and research

What Your Doctor May Not Tell You About PreMenopause

- Dr. John Lee, author
- Good information on irregular/heavy cycles before menopause

What Your Doctor May Not Tell You About Breast Cancer

- Dr. John Lee and Dr. David Zava, authors
- Very detailed, not just about breast cancer, but includes extensive information on hormone metabolism

The Hormone of Desire

- Dr. Susan Rako, author
- About testosterone use in women

Hormone Deception

- D. Lindsey Berkson, author
- About environmental estrogen-like chemicals and their effect on our health

Made in the USA
Middletown, DE
26 April 2019